LOW BACK PAIN:

The Reality Behind the Scans, Surgeries, and Uncertainty

BY GEORGE ACKERMAN, Ph.D., J.D.

ISBN: 979-8995699347 (Paperback Edition)

Dedication

For the past six years, I have dedicated my life to advocating for a cure for Parkinson's disease in memory of my mother and best friend, Sharon. She bravely battled the disease for eighteen years before passing away on January 1, 2020—a loss that changed my life forever.

Since then, I have advocated tirelessly for individuals newly diagnosed with Parkinson's disease and for their families, working to ensure they never feel alone on their journey. In this book, however, I turn inward to confront my own personal struggle—one that has brought its own form of torture and pain: chronic low back pain. My mother also endured severe back pain alongside the many symptoms of Parkinson's disease, a parallel that now feels deeply personal.

This book focuses on my own journey with low back pain, a condition that has often left me debilitated, unable to fully focus on my work or be present with my family. It has cost me time, energy, and participation in the things I care most about—from moments with loved ones to sports, or even the simple ability to wake up without fear that my body may not function that day.

Around the age of forty-two, I woke up one morning and my life was never the same. There was no car accident, traumatic injury, or single defining event. Instead, we believe the cause may be rooted in decades of prolonged sitting—years spent working, studying, earning multiple degrees, completing online coursework, and teaching for long hours at a desk.

This book explores the options I have faced—and continue to face—in search of relief and the ability to function without debilitating low back pain controlling my life. It is a reflection of trial, resilience, frustration, and hope.

This work is dedicated to all those around the world battling chronic low back pain. While our journeys may differ, my hope is that some of the challenges and lessons I have experienced—both negative and positive—may help others feel seen, informed, and less alone. Although chronic low back pain is not a disease, it can still feel endless and overwhelming. It may never be fully cured or completely understood, but there are methods, alternatives, and conversations that deserve attention before life-altering decisions are made—decisions that, without proper information, knowledge, and dialogue, may lead to lasting regret.

Finally, this book is dedicated to my wife, Grether, my best friend and caregiver, who has supported me through surgery and this lifelong journey together; to my children, Brooke, Joshua, and Eli; to my family and friends; and to the global community of individuals battling chronic low back pain. Your unwavering support, understanding, and encouragement have sustained me through this journey and this ongoing battle.

Table of Contents

Chapter 1
Understanding Low Back Pain

Low back pain (LBP) is a widespread condition and one of the leading causes of disability globally. It affects nearly 80% of adults at some point in their lives (Balagué et al., 2012). While often benign and self-limiting, LBP can also indicate serious pathology, making appropriate assessment and management essential.

Epidemiology and Impact

Low back pain is the most common cause of years lived with disability worldwide (Vos et al., 2012). Its lifetime prevalence in adults is estimated to be between 60% and 80% (Hoy et al., 2012). Risk factors include a sedentary lifestyle, obesity, smoking, occupational hazards, and poor posture.

Anatomy of the Low Back

The lumbar spine comprises five vertebrae (L1–L5) supported by intervertebral discs, facet joints, ligaments, muscles, and nerve structures. These components allow for flexibility while bearing the body's weight. Dysfunction in any of these anatomical structures can lead to pain.

Causes of Low Back Pain

A. Mechanical Causes

The most frequent causes are mechanical and include:

- Lumbar strain or sprain
- Degenerative disc disease
- Herniated nucleus pulposus
- Facet joint osteoarthritis
- Spinal stenosis
- Spondylolisthesis

B. Non-Mechanical and Systemic Causes

- Inflammatory: e.g., ankylosing spondylitis
- Infectious: discitis, osteomyelitis
- Neoplastic: primary tumors or metastatic disease
- Referred: from pelvic, renal, or gastrointestinal sources

Classification of Low Back Pain

- Acute: <6 weeks
- Subacute: 6–12 weeks
- Chronic: >12 weeks

Most acute cases resolve within a few weeks; chronic pain often involves psychosocial and functional components requiring multidisciplinary care (Qaseem et al., 2017).

Red Flags in Low Back Pain

Red flags suggest serious underlying disease (Deyo & Weinstein, 2001). These include:

- History of cancer
- Unexplained weight loss
- Fever or systemic symptoms
- Neurological deficits (e.g., saddle anesthesia, incontinence)
- Recent trauma
- Age >50 with new-onset pain

Diagnosis and Evaluation

History and Physical Exam

Assessment focuses on pain characteristics, functional limitations, and neurologic signs. Non-specific LBP (without red flags) rarely requires imaging (Chou et al., 2011).

Diagnostic Imaging and Laboratory Testing

• X-rays: For trauma or structural abnormalities
• MRI: Preferred for neurological deficits or suspected infection/tumor
• CT: Offers detailed bone imaging
• Lab tests: ESR, CRP, CBC in suspected systemic disease

Treatment Strategies

First-Line: Conservative Management

• NSAIDs are more effective than placebo for acute LBP (Qaseem et al., 2017)
• Activity modification: Encourage mobility and discourage bed rest
• Physical therapy: Core strengthening, posture correction
• Heat therapy and manual therapy: May provide symptom relief

Advanced Management

• Epidural steroid injections for radicular pain
• Surgery: Indicated in cases with severe neurological deficits or failure of conservative treatment (e.g., decompression for herniated discs)

Chronic Low Back Pain Management

Multidisciplinary approaches are most effective:

- Cognitive behavioral therapy (CBT) can reduce pain and improve function (Waddell & Burton, 2001)
- Exercise therapy, including yoga and Pilates
- Complementary treatments: spinal manipulation, acupuncture (Sherman et al., 2011)
- Medication: Antidepressants, anti-epileptics; opioids only in select cases with caution (Dowell et al., 2016)

Prevention of Low Back Pain

- Maintain a healthy weight
- Regular exercise focused on core strength
- Proper ergonomics and lifting techniques
- Smoking cessation
- Early management of acute episodes to prevent chronicity

Prognosis

Most patients recover from acute LBP within 4–6 weeks, although recurrence is common. Early intervention and patient education improve long-term outcomes (Waddell & Burton, 2001).

Conclusion

Low back pain remains a major global health concern. While most cases are non-specific and self-limiting, the identification of red flags and use of evidence-based treatment strategies are essential. Prevention through education, lifestyle modification, and early rehabilitation plays a pivotal role in reducing recurrence and disability.

Chapter 2
My Back Journey

I always thought to myself, self...... don't write a book on back pain because people want to hear the better more positive side of results and not needing surgery. Well, here we go anyway!

Pain

I woke up at age 42... I couldn't leave the bed in pain.

10/6/2024....

I was told by a new neurosurgeon that I may still need yet another surgery and that

1) L3-L4 shows disk degeneration, and I would need a disk replacement and
2) The fusion of my SI Joints may not have fused properly

He further discussed the Spine Cord Stimulator which is an advance in technology to hide back pain, but not a solution. However, it can deter me from having a fifth back surgery anytime soon. The decision may be mine, but a very difficult one. I cannot imagine going through another major trauma to my back and mentally it is draining as well.

The Decision. 10/7/2024

I decided to try the SCS. It is not what I want. A tiny pimple or sist bothers me so what will a battery pack installed in me bring? Many say it won't work, some say it does. I am dizzy over the thought of any of this and hoped 4 prior surgeries would have resolved this, but they did not.

Also, this is just to stall the inevitable and likely need for yet a 5th back surgery.

Back Pain and My Journey that Never ends...

I often don't talk about my journey with back pain because to me, losing my mother due to Parkinson's Disease is, was, and will always be the most significant ice-changing event in my life that shifted my life forever towards advocating for a cure for all those battling Pd today in her memory.

Unfortunately, since age 42, I have been battling my medical issues, which I never experienced before age 42, and it just swept up out of nowhere and has indeed destroyed my life.

I lived a life of sports and fitness and never did drugs, but for me, running and playing basketball were my drugs. This changed my life since childhood and helped with my mental health as well as physical health, or so I thought.

I often joke today that doing so much expertise caused my medical issues, but sometimes you cannot win.

As a young child, I was overweight, and around 16, I discovered basketball and fell in love with the sport. I almost slept with a basketball and saw significant changes in my health. Last, I found the gym in college and became a certified personal trainer. I even started my own business, Fitness 4 the Professional, where I trained business professionals throughout South Florida. I also worked as a personal trainer during my master's degree at Gold's Gym and Bally's and thought of becoming a physical therapist and having my gym.

In my personal life, I trained daily and even made it to pass the physical fitness exam for the Federal Bureau of Investigation (FBI) to become a Special Agent, which I later decided to decline for a career in education instead.

I basically lived in the gym throughout my college and Master's career. Facing fitness challenges was a goal of mine; after I met my wife, Grether, we began running in multiple 5Ks for charity and after my mother passed in 2020 for Parkinson's awareness.

Then things changed one Sunday morning; I played basketball with several groups and enjoyed the competition and how I felt during and after I would be on the court for hours. Even when I was a caregiver for my mother, I struggled with stress and depression, and during her battle with PD, I struggled, but when I stepped onto a court, it gave me that short mental break and released something I imagine drugs could provide. A brief escape mentally and physically.

However, on that Sunday, at age 42, I woke up and could not move from my bed. It was a pain in my back that I had never felt before. It was almost like I was having a nightmare, but I was awake. So, I decided to seek medical help, thinking that it was nothing and it likely would pass.

Soon after, and what even today I look back on, was a disaster. I spent hundreds of hours seeking medical help, solutions, and tons of venues to try to combat the pain, from chiropractic to physical therapy, from medicines to back surgeons, from massage therapy too; you name it, I tried it. Before I had never had surgeries except for my ankle, which healed, and I was right back out there doing exercises.

I went to several back doctors who advised me to live with the pain and not to do anymore, but it was easier to say than just suffer silently.

I even tried many different pain management doctors, but medicine was not for me, and after having over 20 injections and minor procedures, I was losing hope. These injections were torture, from epidurals to facet injections to so many I cannot even name them anymore. Still, we exhausted them all, and I was out to sleep so many times, and after, it called nothing but failure, wasting time and high costs for what?

I met a doctor who I will call Dr. S, who I liked him because he made me feel like he could help. So, I had my first back surgery.

Surgery One- Discectomy

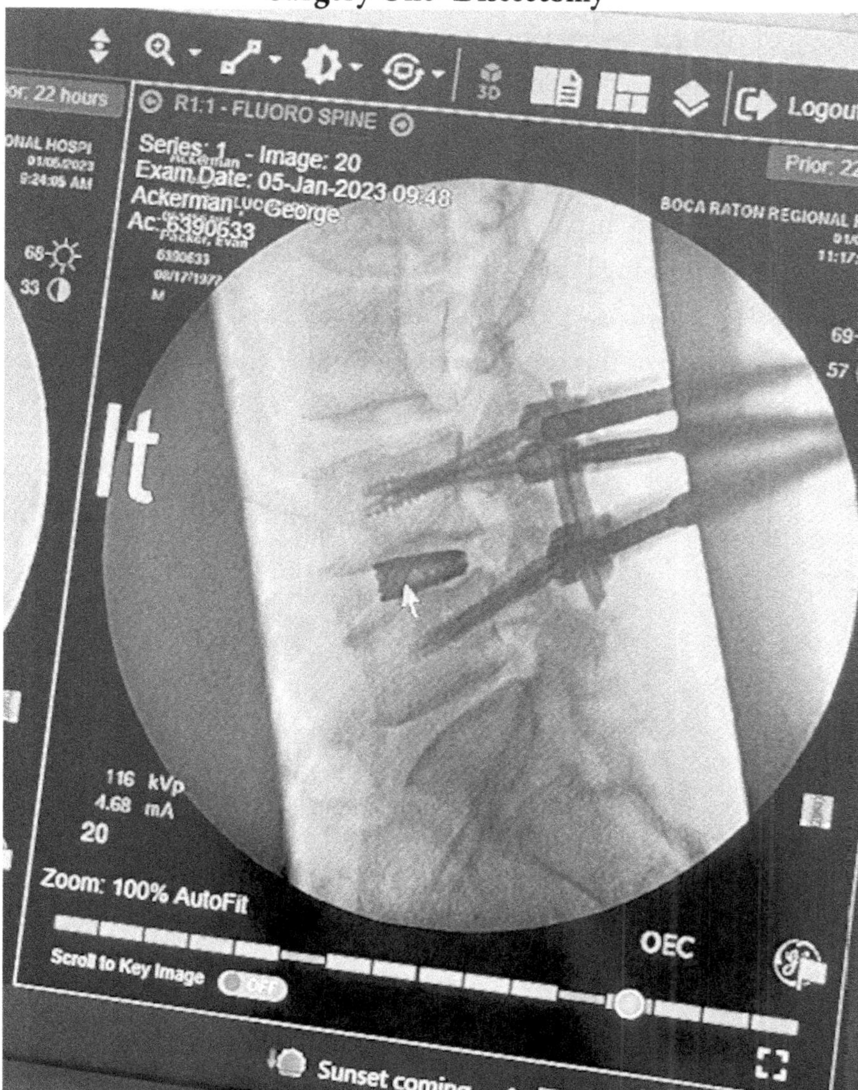

After some time, it did not help. He mentioned a back stimulator, but I was not interested at the time because I didn't understand it and did not even like acne, so I imagined saving a battery would limit my life and make me very uncomfortable.

I then sought a new doctor, Dr P. I truly believed I might make a critical and dangerous decision to move forward with significant surgery, but I prayed that I may have my life back again, I now had three children and an incredible wife who I just wanted to enjoy life again; I always wanted to jog with my daughter and someday travel the world with my wife to England, Spain, France, and Italy, but with the pain, I felt none of this would be possible. So, I continued my journey but turned to potentially life-saving surgery.

Surgery Two

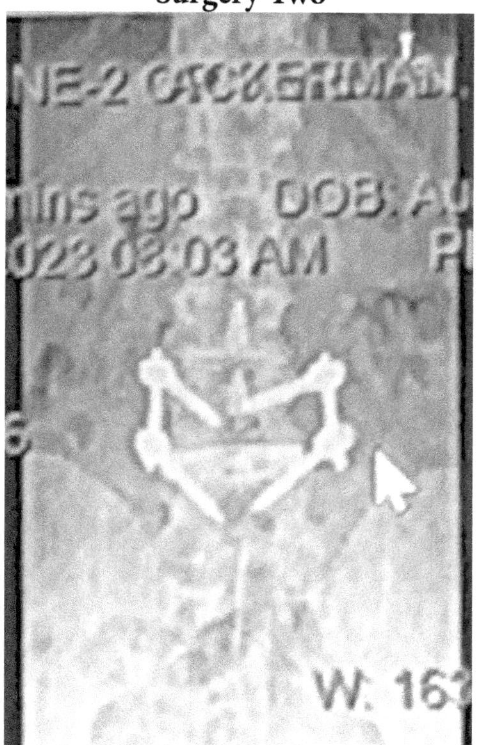

Dr. P embarked on a mission to help me, and I went for surgery for an L4-5 fusion (Surgery with Dr. P)

It was frightening, and the only thing I held onto was hope that this start to a nightmare would end shortly; it did not..... and then I would endure a series of other surgeries to try to correct the pain.

Recovery was tough, and it took months to be able to walk and live again, but the pain continued... intensive therapy and multiple areas to try to rehabilitate. It also felt like a failure.

Surgery Three

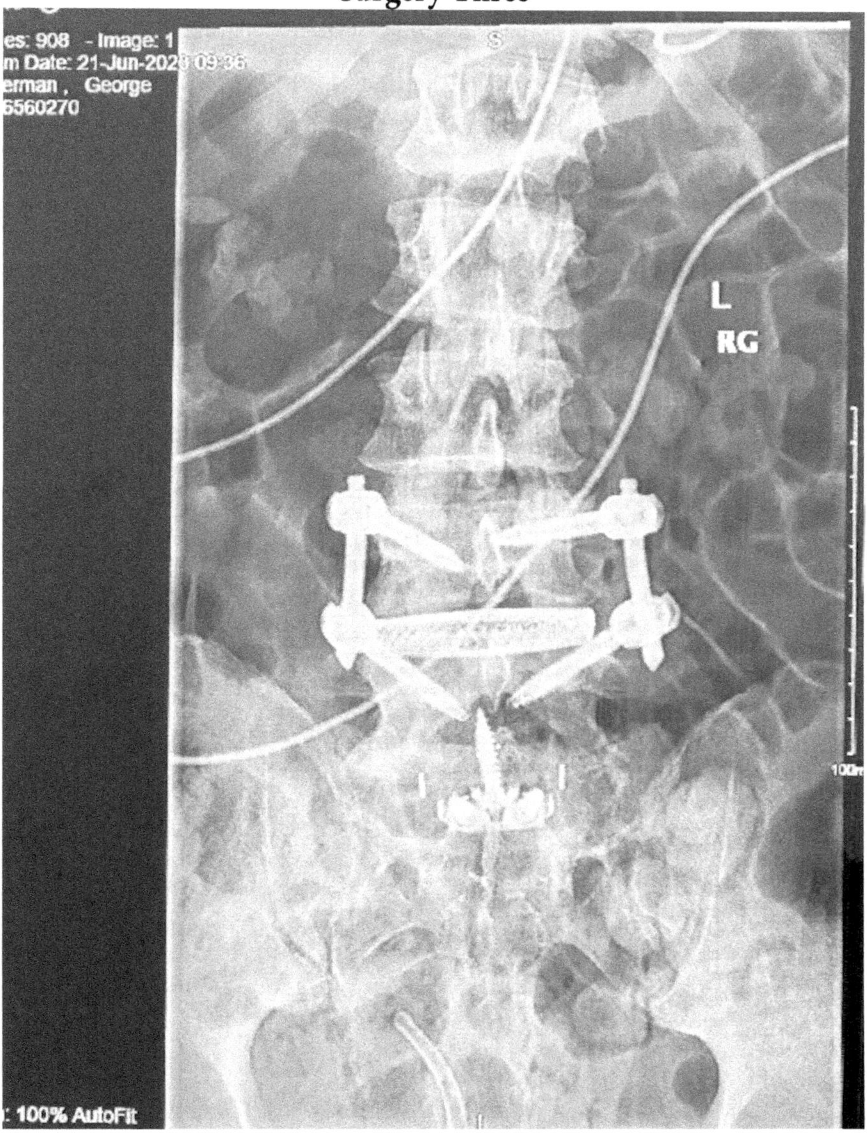

Next was Surgery 3 L5/S1 ALIF (anterior lumbar interbody fusion/ with approach surgeon); L3/4 left hemilaminectomy discectomy.

It did not work. I had temporary help, but it just came back despite this major surgery that put me out for a year. I recall leaving the hospital not knowing the recovery pain that would come next. From the start, on the way home after a two-day stay at the hospital, I needed to walk up a flight of steps at my home to make it to my bed. I made it up the steps but froze and couldn't get through my door in pain. I stood there in shock, crying and screaming in pain. I never experienced any pain like this in my life. It was excruciating, and I felt like breaking down and falling to the floor, but the pain locked my body and mind at that moment, so I pushed through and hoped it wouldn't get any worse.

Meanwhile, my Hospital stay and surgery procedure is another story and chapter for the future; I couldn't describe and share how terrible it was to stay at a hospital and the lousy care I received, or should I say lack of attention received throughout my stay, I am not sure if it was the nurse assigned to me or just reasonable for a hospital in my location. Either way, I do not blame anyone for the back pain.

We had deep discussions and appointments to discuss the next strategy, almost like a national championship in any sport, debating and deciding the next best step.

Surgery Four

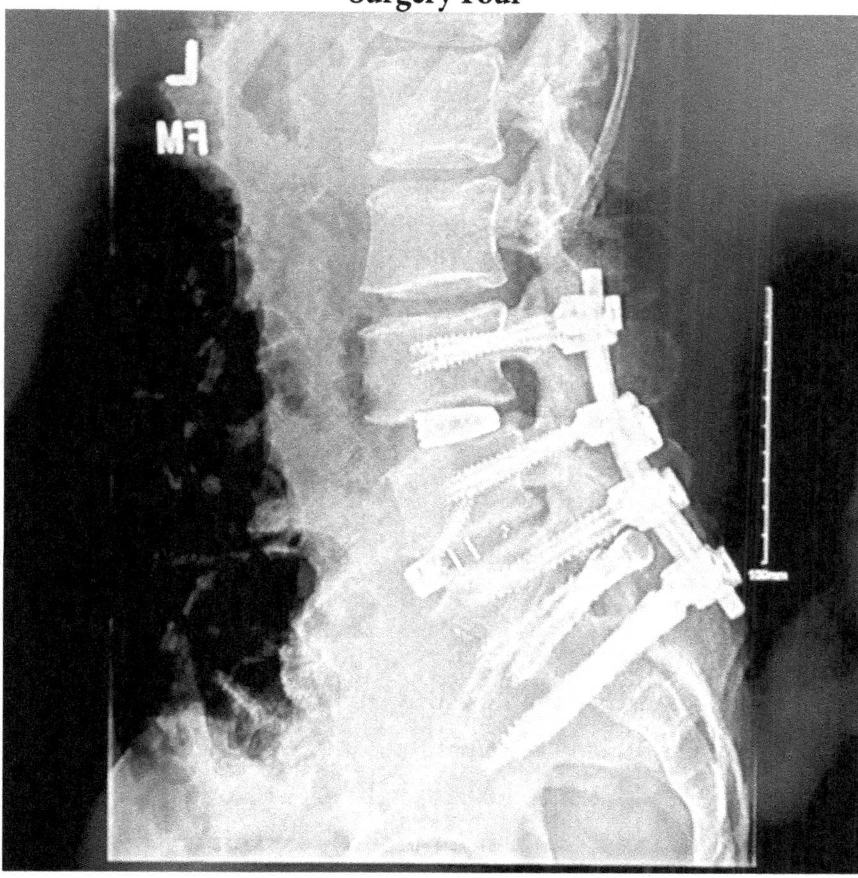

Then came Surgery 4) 6/2024, yet a third major spine surgery to remove items and correct the lowest part of my spine.

Another thing that likely did not work is that today, my lower back has metal and steel in it, which I do, but the feeling of discomfort and pain continues now. The uncomfortable feeling as if there is a metal bar exists day and night because there is hardware that is not allowing me to live or concentrate on life or living,

I have been blessed only to have such a caring and supportive wife who has become a nurse over just a wife these days. I apologized for being in this spot for many years to my wife. I never dreamed I would be like this, but she always provides love, no matter what, and she's there by my side.

The future is uncertain...

So, I lay here typing on **12/16/2024**, heading to a new year, but Santa's of hope and resolution, debating the next step. We discussed likely removing all the back hardware and hoping the fusions worked. If that fails, investigate the spinal cord stimulator, which I know in my heart will not be something I will like, and we do not even know medically if it would work for my situation. So uncertain and more pain to be expected. In addition, removing all the back hardware is dangerous, frightening, and not something I look forward to or even know if should be done.

We put our lives, hope, and future in our medical professionals, not knowing the outcome or if we are making the correct decisions, but ignoring the problem and living in pain is also a horrible alternative.

So, this has continued since age 42, and today, I find myself at age

47, wondering if this is my life here. I am out in multiple doctor's offices, procedures, and surgeries, constantly worrying and wondering if I will ever be able to enjoy life with family or exercise again.

Things could be worse, but they could also be better too. No one deserves this, and I am not sure if finding no resolution somedays is worse than the back pain,

I often wonder if I should share my tales in a book but then figure people want to read the book where you never need surgeons and instead find telling and happier endings where the pain is gone through noninvasive methods, which aren't in the cards in my journey,

So again, writing today, not being able to play sports, no more hope of running with my children, and fear that my future health will limit me from any incredible life experiences now due to my back pain. Even the other night, my wife and daughter were invited to a friend's house for a small gathering, and I was in so much pain I had to decline and stay home alone, resting at age 47. It is unheard of for me because I always enjoyed going out and being social, but I find myself losing the ability to do things like being out because of the constant pain.

So this continues...... sadly in my case, the best may not be yet to come.

Timeline (Only a portion)
My history... of procedures to hide the pain or stop it?

8/7/2025

1st Nerve block, in my middle back but it did not work much.

8/17/21

After the 2nd diagnostic block

My entire low back had no pain. My left thigh, where I had major issues for years, is totally numb. Very successful but not long-lasting.

9/2/21

3rd block, Middle back and upper right side.

9/7/21

I woke up today with my left thigh numb and low back horrible pain only. Feels isolated now only to low back. Upper feels perfect but low is 10/10 pain -- And low back is causing the thigh 100% pain.

9/14/21

Epidural, feel sore.... Not sure if it helped.

9/30/21

A new 2nd doctor initiated Epidural, left thigh felt 100%, back ok, not 100% but little better

Painful procedure.

Lower back bad and middle also—By Friday night the numbness came back in the left thigh. I was relieved for a day or two while I was sleeping woke up at 6 am.

10/7/21

I couldn't leave bed, low back and middle horrible pain, could barely walk, seems to be worse morning.

10/20/21

Today I had low back bad/horrible, left thigh numb.

11/7/21

Back surgery procedure lumbar discectomy. I still feel the thigh pain/numbness

11/11/21

I may need a peripheral nerve surgery https://nevadanervesurgery.org/

11/19

I feel worse. Numb down leg now and back still painful

(2020-2024 4 surgeries-low back pain)

Continued on 2025

6/2025

Epidural worked for 2 days only

7/2025

Another injection, a new pain management Doctor.

My Journal

5/27/21 First visit Dr B. The thigh pain shifted to the right side of the left thigh but more of a pulling feeling, low back pain also

5/28/21 Back sore after injection, feels odd but no pain, thigh perfect

5/29 Upper left side back pain (uncomfortable like a knot), next to shoulder blade one side

5/31 Back pain bad, didn't sleep, thigh no pain, need pain medicine

6/1 Same back pain, not as bad, thigh no pain

6/2 and 6/3 Ran, less back pain, no thigh pain

6/6 Still thigh 100% no pain, back horrible pain though

6/7 Monday Back bad, thigh fine

6/8 Top of back pain, low back also pain.

First shots- back pain existed, thigh pain left for 1 week.

Second Shots- -Back/thigh seem worse after second shots? Back (upper, middle and lower pain) Thigh, fully back with full pain.

6/8/21 I saw a pain management doctor- injections (3 to back)

Nighttime my left thigh is numb, back and itching again.

6/9/21 I didn't sleep-top back pain uncomfortable

Daytime-thigh burning again

The upper left and right under shoulder blade are new pain

6/10/21 Back pain back 24/7, constant all day bothered me while working. Sitting, legs and foot pain also (never had foot before) throbbing

Sitting was tough all day

EVENING - no pain, worked out, though was odd but ok

*** Woke up at 5am thigh burning badly, all back again

6/11/21 Seeing chiropractor today. Ran in the morning- felt pain but bearable.

Back from Chiro. Feel much, much happier and better. Hope may return now. Chiropractor Dr WM

6/12/21 Had a massage, 1 hour, feel ok today,

Followed chiropractor directions used cold ice, 15 min stimulator, and did exercises provided (3 knee to stomach, turkey neck and shoulder movement)

6/13/21 I woke up to horrible pain everywhere, though, back upper, middle and back, like someone punched me in the back and chest (felt odd breathing also) like it is all attached somehow) When I breath the back hurts all over top to bottom

6/14/21 I woke up in pain, just lay down hurts-low back.

Walking around painfully. I took vitamins for my back, did cold ice, tens unit, exercises chiro said but still worse.

Used ice, stimulation all day (helps while using but not after I stop it)

************** First time feet felt throbbing, Feet, felt like blood rushing though no pain but very odd and uncomfortable

I woke up around 3 am and didn't sleep again.....

Pain during nighttime. Middle back hurts but prior to shots it was only the lower back and now it feels like it is the entire back. Trouble breathing because pressing that area of the back. Never had this pain prior to back injections.

Awake the entire night. Middle of back. Trouble laying down, trouble breathing, cannot sleep or lay back down. Never had this prior to injections.

I stay awake staring at the wall wondering if this is how the rest of my life will be in pain permanently and where it came from and why. I'm not sure if the bed is an issue or pillow but this never hurt prior to injections.

By 4:30 am I tried sleeping with an ice pack not on low back but for upper back left side under shoulder blade and middle back both sides horribly uncomfortable around 10 pain. Prevented me from sleeping all night. Ice ok but still couldn't sleep.

Injections are not helping just making other portions of back worsen specifically feels like my back is stabbed mid-section opposite to heart and trouble each time breathe. Plus, the upper left back under the shoulder blade is extremely painful.

I never had prior to injections where original pain was low back. It feels like pain spread worse.

I'm not sure what to do next and have no pain medicine for emergencies so I stayed awake the entire night. Earlier feet throbbing went away.

6/15/21 Sitting for work hurts now/pain. The first time seems it is pain day and night, no relief at all.

I went to a stretch Zone, and it felt good. I had hope and called my general dr who prescribed two medicines for the pain. General Dr stated see physical therapy and *prescribed meloxicam and cyclobenzaprine* for pain.

6/16/21 I was excited maybe it would work but woke up at 4 am with horrible pain in the left middle/upper back. This pain wasn't the original low back pain. It seems to be from the shots, and I cannot breathe comfortably and seems the original pain shifted and is in a worse spot, so this continues.

6/17/21 Morning middle back left side pain, used a (lidocaine) patch and ok there on out

Thigh Itching

6/18/21 Thigh itching all night, wore up 2, back uncomfortable/pain

6/19/21 I felt uncomfortable pain throughout entire back. Used the tens unit, heating pad for twenty minutes. Itching left thigh, but no pain. It's not easy to live like this though and can't exercise or do any normal routine anymore. Not using the low back stretching machine again seems to have caused more pain.

6/20/21 I woke up with tons of pain in back and thigh burning again. Seems to be back at the same place in pain as 3 weeks ago.

6/21/21 No pain today, at all. I saw a physical therapist using the stretch machine on the floor for 15 min.

6/22/21 Feel ok... taking for 3 weeks (relief factor vitamins)

> Epimedium (Aerial-goat weed) – 200 mg
> Turmeric (Rhizome longa L.) – 667 mg
> Japanese Fleeceflower (Root/Resveratrol) – 70 mg
> EPA (Eicosapentaenoic Acid/omega 3 fish oil) – 647 mg
> DHA (Docosahexaenoic Acid) – 253 mg

Saw Doctor EP and MD Surgeon who stated surgery not needed yet.

6/28/21 I woke up in horrible low back pain, thigh ok, from playing basketball. I went to the chiro and after my visit it was no pain. However, it seems to come back a day later.

9/21- 11/21 I continued seeing medical professionals, physical therapy and stretching did not help. INJECTIONS WITH Dr. *GZ (Pain Mgt)*

I went to the pain management doctor for months, have several injections. It all helped temporarily but low back pain came back.

9/14/21, 9/7/21, 9/2/21, 8/23/21, 8/11/21, 8/5/217/26/21 (Visits)

<u>Around 1/2022 went to Dr S (Surgeon) and Dr M (pain management)</u>

1/14/22 2nd MRI/CT Scan

4/2022 Dr S did a Lumbar Discectomy which helped the left thigh pain 100%, but it did not help the low back pain at all but was not supposed to help the back.

3/2022 I tried back relief program vitamins (did not help) and multiple drugs (did not help)

Medicines tried:

Meloxicam 15 MG
Celeoxib 200 MG
Cyclobenzaprine 10 MG

5/2022 I had an epidural, 2 additional sets of injections..... did not help

6/1/2022 I did a Radio Frequency Ablation.... It did not help.

6/27/22 I started Acupuncture

6/28/22 I started with a new physical therapist

7/1/22-9/19/22

Tried acupuncture
Intense physical therapy
Intense personal training
Intense massage/laser
Medicines do not work
Read books on it, exercises, yoga, nothing works more than a night.

Used Ice all day, heat all night, special bed, standing desk, nothing is working more than a night to relieve the pain

Everything feels good that night and then next day back to pain

9/20/22 Called Dr EP (Surgeon) for follow up.

I had a CT scan and 2 MRI's and discussed 11/2/22 a Spinal Fusion: Lateral Lumbar Interbody Fusion (LLIF)

1/1/23 I woke up at 4 am and couldn't move, I'm not sure if the area is the L4-L5 but I documented with a photo.

1/7/22 Fusion Surgery L4-L5 Dr P. SURGERY 1

Horrible pain after, we would see if it worked...

5/2/23 I still have pain, fusion helped 10% but did not solve my issue,

6/20/23 L5/S1 ALIF (anterior lumbar interbody fusion/ with approach surgeon); L3/4 left hemilaminectomy discectomy with Dr P. SURGERY 2

8/1/2023 Through 5/1/2024 I am still experiencing pain 24/7 but isolated to the left, middle and right waistline where I would wear a belt. I even investigated the stimulator to be inserted for pain but decided to do 1 final surgery first.

I went to another pain management dr, 2 epidurals, nothing helped.

5/2124 I went back for a third and hopefully final spine surgery. Revision and removal of hardware/instrumentation L4, L5 Posterior Fusion/instrumentation L-S2. PACKER SURGERY 3

2024 to 2026 many more procedures and medical visits not documented in my journal. The Journey continues at no end it seems....

Chapter 3
The Science- Low Back Pain

Introduction

Low back pain (LBP) is one of the most common musculoskeletal conditions globally, affecting individuals across all age groups and socioeconomic statuses. It is a leading cause of disability and work absenteeism, with a significant impact on healthcare systems and individual quality of life (Hartvigsen et al., 2018). This chapter provides an overview of the epidemiology, risk factors, pathophysiology, clinical presentation, diagnosis, and evidence-based management strategies for low back pain.

Epidemiology

Low back pain is a pervasive health issue, with an estimated lifetime prevalence of 60% to 80% (Balagué et al., 2012). According to the Global Burden of Disease Study, LBP is the leading cause of years lived with disability worldwide (GBD 2017 Disease and Injury Incidence and Prevalence Collaborators, 2018). It most commonly affects individuals between the ages of 30 and 50 and is slightly more prevalent in women than men.

Risk Factors

Numerous factors contribute to the development of low back pain, including:

- Physical factors: Poor posture, manual labor, heavy lifting, and prolonged sitting.
- Psychosocial factors: Depression, anxiety, and job dissatisfaction (Pincus et al., 2002).
- Lifestyle factors: Obesity, smoking, and sedentary behavior (Shiri et al., 2010).

These factors often interact in complex ways, making the etiology of LBP multifactorial and individualized.

Pathophysiology

LBP can be classified as acute (<6 weeks), subacute (6–12 weeks), or chronic (>12 weeks). Most cases are nonspecific, meaning no clear pathoanatomical cause can be identified. Common anatomical sources include muscles, ligaments, intervertebral discs, and facet joints (Maher et al., 2017).

Specific causes, such as herniated discs, spinal stenosis, or vertebral fractures, are less common but require targeted diagnostic and therapeutic approaches. Inflammatory or systemic diseases (e.g., ankylosing spondylitis or metastatic cancer) should also be ruled out in cases presented with red flags.

Clinical Presentation

Patients with low back pain typically report localized pain in the lumbar region, which may be accompanied by stiffness, limited mobility, or radiation to the buttocks or legs. Neurological symptoms such as numbness or weakness suggest nerve root involvement and warrant further investigation (Chou et al., 2016).

Red flags indicating possible serious underlying pathology include:

- History of trauma
- Unexplained weight loss
- Fever
- History of cancer
- Immunosuppression
- Night pain or pain at rest
- Saddle anesthesia or bladder dysfunction

Diagnosis

For most patients, a detailed history and physical examination are sufficient for diagnosis. Imaging is not routinely recommended unless red flags are present or if symptoms persist beyond 6 weeks despite conservative treatment (Qaseem et al., 2017).

• X-rays can identify fractures or structural abnormalities.
• MRI is useful for evaluating soft tissues and detecting disc herniation or spinal tumors.
• CT scans offer detailed bone imaging and may be considered when MRI is contraindicated.

Management

Acute Low Back Pain

Most cases of acute LBP resolve within a few weeks. Management focuses on:

• Education and reassurance
• Maintaining activity levels
• Short-term pharmacologic therapy, such as NSAIDs
(Deyo et al., 2015)

Bed rest is discouraged, and early return to normal activities is associated with faster recovery.

Chronic Low Back Pain

Management of chronic LBP is multifaceted and may include:

• Physical therapy: Exercise programs improve function and reduce pain.
• Cognitive-behavioral therapy (CBT): Helps address maladaptive

beliefs and behaviors (Henschke et al., 2010).
• Pharmacologic treatments: Includes NSAIDs, muscle relaxants, or in select cases, antidepressants and opioids (used cautiously).
• Interventional procedures: Such as spinal injections, considered in refractory cases.
• Multidisciplinary rehabilitation: Combining physical, psychological, and vocational interventions has shown the best outcomes (Kamper et al., 2015).

Prevention

Preventive strategies include promoting physical activity, ergonomic education, and addressing psychosocial risk factors in the workplace. Evidence supports that regular exercise and maintaining a healthy weight can reduce the risk of recurrent LBP (Steffens et al., 2016).

Conclusion

Low back pain is a common, multifactorial condition with significant implications for individuals and society. While most cases are benign and self-limiting, appropriate evaluation and evidence-based management are crucial to improving outcomes and preventing chronicity. Continued research into the biopsychosocial mechanisms of LBP is essential for developing innovative interventions and improving patient care.

Chapter 4
Causes of Low Back Pain

Low back pain (LBP) is one of the most prevalent musculoskeletal disorders worldwide and a leading cause of disability across all age groups (Wu et al., 2020). It is a multifactorial condition influenced by a variety of anatomical, mechanical, lifestyle, and psychosocial factors. Understanding the causes of low back pain is essential for clinicians and patients alike, as it informs both prevention strategies and treatment plans. This chapter provides a comprehensive overview of the primary and contributing causes of low back pain, categorizing them into mechanical, degenerative, traumatic, systemic, and psychosocial origins.

Mechanical and Postural Causes

Mechanical causes are the most common source of low back pain, often resulting from abnormal stress on spinal structures such as muscles, ligaments, intervertebral discs, and facet joints (Maher et al., 2017). Poor posture, repetitive movements, improper lifting techniques, and prolonged sitting can contribute to muscle strain or ligament sprain, leading to acute or chronic low back pain. For example, slouching while sitting can increase lumbar spine pressure, promoting disc degeneration over time.

Additionally, physical deconditioning due to sedentary behavior can lead to weakness in core and back muscles, exacerbating postural imbalance and increasing vulnerability to injury (Adams et al., 2020). Improper ergonomics at the workplace is also a significant contributor to mechanical back pain, particularly among office workers and individuals in occupations requiring heavy lifting.

Degenerative Causes

Age-related degeneration is another leading cause of low back pain. Degenerative disc disease (DDD) occurs when intervertebral discs lose hydration and elasticity, decreasing their ability to absorb mechanical loads. This can result in disc bulging, herniation, or narrowing of the spinal canal (spinal stenosis) (Brinjikji et al., 2015). Degenerative changes in the facet joints, known as facet arthropathy, can also cause localized low back pain and stiffness.

Osteoarthritis, commonly affecting older adults, contributes to spinal degeneration, leading to pain, reduced mobility, and inflammation. Spondylolisthesis, a condition in which one vertebra slips over another, is often the result of degeneration and can cause nerve compression and radiating pain into the lower extremities.

Traumatic and Injury-Related Causes

Trauma to the lumbar spine, such as that resulting from falls, car accidents, or sports injuries, can lead to acute low back pain. Fractures, ligamentous injuries, and disc herniation are common outcomes of significant spinal trauma. Even minor injuries, if recurrent or untreated, may lead to chronic pain syndromes (Deyo & Mirza, 2016).

Athletes and physically active individuals are at increased risk of overuse injuries, particularly stress fractures in the pars interarticularis, which may lead to spondylolysis and subsequent spondylolisthesis (Standaert & Herring, 2007).

Systemic and Pathological Causes

Although less common, systemic conditions can also cause low back pain. These include inflammatory diseases such as ankylosing spondylitis, infections like vertebral osteomyelitis, and neoplastic conditions including spinal metastases. These causes are often characterized by a constant, non-mechanical type of pain that does not improve with rest (Hartvigsen et al., 2018).

Red flag symptoms such as unexplained weight loss, night pain, or a history of cancer should prompt clinicians to investigate serious underlying conditions.

Psychosocial and Behavioral Factors

Recent research highlights the biopsychosocial nature of low back pain. Psychological stress, depression, anxiety, and poor coping mechanisms are strongly associated with both the onset and persistence of low back pain (Pinheiro et al., 2016). Individuals experiencing psychological distress may have a heightened perception of pain or altered pain processing, which exacerbates their symptoms and complicates recovery.

Social factors such as job dissatisfaction, low social support, and disability compensation claims have also been identified as risk factors for chronic low back pain (Foster et al., 2018). These findings underscore the need for a holistic approach to diagnosis and management.

Conclusion

The causes of low back pain are diverse and often multifactorial, ranging from mechanical and degenerative to systemic and psychosocial origins. Effective diagnosis and treatment depend on a thorough understanding of these etiologies and their interactions. Healthcare providers should adopt a comprehensive, individualized approach to patient care, incorporating physical, psychological, and social assessments to address the root causes of low back pain and improve patient outcomes.

Chapter 5
Diagnosis and Evaluation

Low back pain (LBP) is one of the most prevalent musculoskeletal complaints globally and a leading cause of disability across all age groups. Accurate diagnosis and thorough evaluation are essential to identify the underlying cause and guide effective management. This chapter explores the diagnostic approach, including clinical evaluation, imaging, and differential diagnosis, in accordance with evidence-based guidelines.

Clinical History and Physical Examination

The first and most critical step in evaluating low back pain is a detailed patient history. Clinicians must assess the onset, duration, character, and aggravating or relieving factors of the pain. Important "red flags" such as unexplained weight loss, fever, history of cancer, recent trauma, or neurological deficits may suggest serious underlying pathology, such as malignancy, infection, or spinal fracture (Qaseem et al., 2017).

The physical examination complements the history and typically includes assessment of posture, gait, spinal range of motion, and a neurologic exam to evaluate reflexes, motor strength, and sensation. Special tests, such as the straight-leg raise (SLR) test, can help identify radiculopathy due to lumbar disc herniation (Deyo & Weinstein, 2001).

Classification of Low Back Pain

Low back pain can be classified into three broad categories: nonspecific low back pain, radicular pain (commonly due to nerve root compression), and pain associated with specific spinal pathology. The vast majority (over 85%) of cases fall into the nonspecific category, where no definitive cause can be identified (Chou et al., 2007).

Radiculopathy is suspected when there is leg pain in a dermatomal distribution, often accompanied by motor or sensory changes. Specific spinal pathology includes conditions such as spinal stenosis, vertebral compression fractures, infections, or tumors. A precise diagnosis in these cases is vital for prompt intervention.

Role of Imaging

Routine imaging is not recommended in the initial evaluation of nonspecific low back pain due to its low diagnostic yield and the risk of incidental findings leading to unnecessary interventions. Imaging should be reserved for patients with severe or progressive neurological deficits or when red flags are present (Qaseem et al., 2017).

When indicated, plain radiography may be used to detect fractures or severe degenerative changes. Magnetic resonance imaging (MRI) is the preferred modality for evaluating soft tissue, nerve roots, and spinal cord structures and is highly sensitive for detecting infections, tumors, and disc herniations (Jarvik & Deyo, 2002). Computed tomography (CT) can be helpful in visualizing bony structures when MRI is contraindicated.

Laboratory Evaluation

Although not routinely required, laboratory tests such as erythrocyte sedimentation rate (ESR), C-reactive protein (CRP), and complete blood count (CBC) may be warranted if an infectious or inflammatory cause is suspected. Elevated markers of inflammation can point toward conditions like spinal osteomyelitis or ankylosing spondylitis (Ropper & Zafonte, 2015).

Differential Diagnosis

A thorough evaluation should consider multiple potential causes. Mechanical causes, such as muscle strain, degenerative disc disease, or spondylolisthesis, are common. Systemic conditions like metastatic cancer or infections must also be considered, particularly in older adults or immunocompromised patients. Referred pain from visceral sources, such as pancreatitis or renal colic, can also mimic LBP and must be included in the differential diagnosis.

Conclusion

The diagnosis and evaluation of low back pain require a structured and evidence-based approach. Most cases can be managed conservatively with reassurance and physical therapy, but timely identification of serious pathology is critical. A comprehensive clinical assessment, supported by judicious use of imaging and laboratory tests, ensures accurate diagnosis and guides appropriate treatment planning.

Chapter 6
Alternatives to Back Surgery

Low back pain (LBP) remains one of the most common musculoskeletal complaints globally, with significant implications for individual well-being and public health. While surgical interventions are sometimes necessary, particularly in cases involving severe spinal deformity, nerve compression, or failed conservative care, a majority of patients can benefit from non-surgical treatments. Understanding alternatives to surgery is essential in fostering informed decision-making, optimizing outcomes, and reducing healthcare costs.

Conservative Management Approaches
Physical Therapy

Physical therapy (PT) is a cornerstone of conservative care for LBP. Exercise-based interventions, including strengthening, flexibility, and aerobic conditioning, have been shown to improve function and reduce pain (Qaseem et al., 2017). Therapists often employ a combination of manual therapy, postural education, and core stabilization to address biomechanical dysfunction.

Cognitive functional therapy (CFT), an advanced form of PT, integrates behavioral strategies with movement retraining and has shown promise for chronic low back pain (O'Sullivan et al., 2015).

Pharmacological Management

Nonsteroidal anti-inflammatory drugs (NSAIDs), muscle relaxants, and in some cases, short-term opioids may be used to manage pain and inflammation (Deyo et al., 2015). However, medications are ideally used as part of a broader treatment plan, with attention to the risks of long-term use and dependency, particularly with opioids.

Chiropractic and Osteopathic Manipulation

Spinal manipulation, typically performed by chiropractors or osteopathic physicians, is a commonly used intervention. Studies suggest that for some patients with acute or subacute LBP, spinal manipulation may provide moderate relief (Paige et al., 2017). While the exact mechanisms remain debated, neurophysiological and mechanical effects likely contribute to its efficacy.

Acupuncture

Acupuncture, a traditional Chinese medicine modality, has gained popularity as an alternative therapy for LBP. Systematic reviews indicate it may reduce pain and improve function, especially when combined with conventional treatments (Vickers et al., 2018). While not universally accepted, acupuncture is generally considered safe when performed by trained professionals.

Behavioral and Psychological Interventions

Cognitive Behavioral Therapy (CBT)

Psychological factors significantly influence pain perception and disability in chronic LBP. CBT focuses on modifying maladaptive thoughts and behaviors associated with pain. Clinical trials demonstrate that CBT can significantly reduce pain intensity, improve mood, and enhance quality of life in patients with chronic low back pain (Ehde et al., 2014).

Mindfulness-Based Stress Reduction (MBSR)

MBSR incorporates meditation, yoga, and body awareness and has shown beneficial effects for chronic pain syndromes, including LBP. A landmark study by Cherkin et al. (2016) found that MBSR was as effective as CBT and superior to usual care in improving function and pain outcomes.

Interventional Procedures

Epidural Steroid Injections (ESIs)

ESIs are commonly used for radicular pain due to disc herniation or spinal stenosis. While effective for short-term relief, their long-term benefit is questionable (Chou et al., 2015). ESIs can serve as a bridge for patients attempting rehabilitation or delaying surgery.

Radiofrequency Ablation (RFA)

RFA targets the medial branch nerves that supply facet joints and has been found to provide prolonged pain relief in appropriately selected patients (Cohen et al., 2020). This procedure is particularly useful for patients with confirmed facet-mediated pain and no neurological deficits.

Lifestyle and Self-Management Strategies

Patient education and self-care play a pivotal role in LBP management. Encouraging patients to remain active, avoid bed rest, and maintain a healthy lifestyle are all core recommendations. Smoking cessation, weight loss, and ergonomic modifications also contribute to long-term improvements (Qaseem et al., 2017).

Multidisciplinary Pain Programs

Multidisciplinary pain management combines medical, physical, and psychological therapies. These programs address the biopsychosocial aspects of chronic LBP and have demonstrated greater effectiveness than standard care or surgery in many cases (Gatchel et al., 2014). They are particularly beneficial for patients with complex or refractory pain.

Conclusion

While surgery may be indicated for specific structural pathologies, the vast majority of patients with low back pain can benefit from non-surgical interventions. A multimodal, individualized approach—integrating physical, pharmacological, psychological, and interventional treatments—often yield optimal outcomes. Patient education, shared decision-making, and ongoing evaluation are essential to effective management and avoidance of unnecessary surgical procedures.

Chapter 7
Spinal Cord Stimulator

Chronic pain is a debilitating condition affecting millions worldwide, often persisting despite conservative treatments. One advanced intervention gaining traction in pain management is the spinal cord stimulator (SCS). Originally developed in the 1960s, SCS has evolved significantly, offering a minimally invasive option to manage refractory pain, particularly in cases of failed back surgery syndrome (FBSS), complex regional pain syndrome (CRPS), and chronic low back or limb pain. This chapter explores the mechanisms, indications, procedure, efficacy, risks, and future directions of spinal cord stimulation in modern medicine.

Mechanism of Action

The spinal cord stimulator delivers mild electrical impulses to the dorsal columns of the spinal cord through implanted electrodes, modulating pain signals before they reach the brain. This process is based on the gate control theory of pain, where non-painful input closes the nerve "gates" to painful input, effectively reducing the perception of pain (Melzack & Wall, 1965). By altering neural activity in the spinal cord, SCS can reduce both the intensity and unpleasantness of pain.

Indications for Use

SCS is typically considered after the failure of more conservative measures such as physical therapy, medications, and less invasive procedures. Key indications include:

- Failed Back Surgery Syndrome (FBSS)
- Complex Regional Pain Syndrome (CRPS)
- Peripheral neuropathy
- Chronic intractable angina
- Painful diabetic neuropathy

Careful patient selection, based on psychological screening and successful trial stimulation, is essential for optimal outcomes (Kumar et al., 2007).

The Procedure

The implantation of an SCS system occurs in two stages:

1. Trial Phase: A temporary electrode is inserted percutaneously under fluoroscopic guidance, and an external pulse generator is used. The patient typically undergoes a 3–7-day trial to assess pain relief.
2. Permanent Implantation: If the trial is successful (commonly

defined as at least 50% pain relief), a permanent system is implanted. This includes electrodes and a pulse generator surgically placed under the skin, typically in the buttock or abdomen.

Modern systems allow for rechargeable batteries and the use of wireless programming via patient-controlled remotes or mobile applications.

Efficacy and Outcomes

Numerous studies confirm the effectiveness of SCS in reducing chronic pain and improving quality of life. A landmark randomized trial by Kumar et al. (2007) demonstrated superior outcomes for SCS combined with conventional medical management versus conventional management alone in FBSS patients. Long-term studies show sustained pain relief and improved functional outcomes in well-selected patients (North et al., 2011).

However, efficacy may decrease over time in some patients due to lead migration, scar tissue formation, or adaptation to stimulation. Advances such as high-frequency stimulation and burst stimulation aim to overcome these limitations by providing pain relief without paresthesia.

Risks and Complications

While SCS is generally safe, potential complications include:

- Lead migration or breakage
- Infection at the implant site

- Cerebrospinal fluid leak
- Hardware malfunction
- Pain at the implant site

Proper surgical technique and patient education are critical to minimizing these risks (Deer et al., 2014).

Psychological Considerations

Psychological evaluation is a crucial component of patient selection. Patients with untreated psychiatric disorders, poor coping mechanisms, or unrealistic expectations may have poorer outcomes (Block et al., 2001). Cognitive behavioral therapy and counseling may be recommended before or during SCS treatment to improve coping skills and outcomes.

Advances and Future Directions

Technological advancements are transforming SCS therapy. Novel developments include:

- High-frequency stimulation (10 kHz): Provides pain relief without paresthesia.
- Closed-loop systems: Adjust stimulation based on feedback from spinal cord activity.
- MRI-compatible devices: Allow for safer imaging.
- Bluetooth and mobile app integration: Enhance user control and remote programming.

Research into individualized neuromodulation patterns and integration with wearable technologies is ongoing, holding promise for improved patient-specific outcomes.

Conclusion

Spinal cord stimulation is a powerful tool in the management of chronic pain, particularly for patients unresponsive to other treatments. With continuous technological innovation and improved patient selection criteria, SCS offers hope and enhanced quality of life for individuals suffering from long-term, intractable pain. As research progresses, the future of neuromodulation in pain management continues to brighten.

Chapter 8
The Last Resort- Surgical Intervention for Low Back Pain

Low back pain (LBP) is a widespread condition affecting individuals globally, with significant socioeconomic impacts. While most cases of LBP resolve with conservative management, a subset of patients experience persistent, debilitating symptoms that may warrant surgical intervention. Surgical procedures for low back pain are typically considered when non-surgical treatments have failed and specific structural abnormalities—such as herniated discs, spinal stenosis, or spondylolisthesis—are present. This chapter provides an overview of the indications, types, outcomes, and risks of surgical procedures used to treat low back pain.

Indications for Surgery

Surgical intervention for LBP is generally reserved for cases where conservative therapies—including physical therapy, medications, and injections—have not provided adequate relief over an extended period (typically 6–12 weeks). Common surgical indications include:

- Disc herniation causing nerve root compression with radiculopathy
- Spinal stenosis leading to neurogenic claudication
- Spondylolisthesis with instability or nerve involvement
- Degenerative disc disease with severe, disabling pain
- Spinal deformities such as scoliosis or kyphosis
- Failed back surgery syndrome requiring revision procedures

Surgical decision-making should be individualized, incorporating imaging findings, clinical symptoms, and patient preferences (Chou et al., 2009).

Common Surgical Procedures

1. Discectomy and Microdiscectomy

A discectomy involves removing part or all of a herniated disc pressing on a spinal nerve. A microdiscectomy, a minimally invasive version of the procedure, uses a smaller incision and microscopic visualization, reducing tissue damage and recovery time (Weinstein et al., 2006).

2. Laminectomy

Laminectomy involves the removal of part of the vertebral bone called the lamina to relieve pressure on the spinal cord or nerves, often used to treat spinal stenosis. The procedure may be performed with or without spinal fusion, depending on spinal stability (Deyo et al., 2010).

3. Spinal Fusion

Spinal fusion is used to stabilize the spine by permanently joining two or more vertebrae. It is indicated for degenerative disc disease, spondylolisthesis, or instability. Despite its frequency, the efficacy of spinal fusion for chronic low back pain remains controversial (Brox et al., 2003; Fritzell et al., 2001).

4. Artificial Disc Replacement

Disc replacement is an alternative to fusion that aims to preserve motion at the spinal segment. It may reduce adjacent segment disease compared to fusion, though long-term outcomes are still being evaluated (Guyer et al., 2009).

Outcomes and Effectiveness

Surgical outcomes vary based on the procedure, patient characteristics, and underlying pathology. Generally, patients with radicular symptoms due to disc herniation or stenosis experience better outcomes than those with nonspecific chronic back pain. The SPORT trial showed that patients undergoing surgery for herniated discs and stenosis had better pain relief and functional outcomes than those treated non-surgically (Weinstein et al., 2006; 2008).

However, outcomes for spinal fusion in degenerative disc disease are less predictable, and benefits may not significantly exceed those of intensive rehabilitation (Fairbank et al., 2005).

Risks and Complications

Surgical treatment carries potential complications, including:

- Infection
- Bleeding
- Nerve injury
- Hardware failure
- Adjacent segment disease
- Persistent or recurrent pain (failed back surgery syndrome)

Reoperation rates vary by procedure but may be as high as 10–20% within five years (Martin et al., 2007). Proper patient selection and preoperative counseling are critical to minimize risks and optimize outcomes.

Conclusion

Surgery for low back pain can offer significant relief for carefully selected patients with clear anatomical causes of symptoms. Procedures like microdiscectomy and laminectomy tend to have favorable outcomes, especially for radiculopathy and spinal stenosis. However, spinal fusion remains controversial for nonspecific back pain due to variable results. Shared decision-making, evidence-based guidelines, and patient-centered care are essential to guide surgical treatment decisions in low back pain.

Chapter 9
Treatment

Low back pain (LBP) is one of the most common musculoskeletal disorders worldwide, affecting people of all ages and socioeconomic statuses. It is a leading cause of disability and contributes significantly to healthcare costs, lost productivity, and reduced quality of life (Hartvigsen et al., 2018). Effective management of low back pain requires a multimodal approach that incorporates both non-invasive and, in some cases, surgical interventions. The treatment strategy is largely determined by the underlying cause, severity, and duration of symptoms, as well as patient preferences and comorbidities.

Conservative Treatments
Physical Therapy and Exercise

Physical therapy is a cornerstone of LBP treatment, particularly in cases of nonspecific or chronic pain. Therapeutic exercise improves mobility, strengthens the core muscles, and helps restore function (Qaseem et al., 2017). Modalities such as stretching, aerobic conditioning, and stabilization exercises are commonly employed. Studies show that supervised exercise therapy is more effective than rest or passive modalities alone in improving pain and function (Foster et al., 2018).

Pharmacologic Interventions

Medications are frequently used to manage pain, especially in the acute phase. Nonsteroidal anti-inflammatory drugs (NSAIDs) are typically the first-line pharmacologic treatment due to their effectiveness in reducing inflammation and pain (van Tulder et al., 2006). Muscle relaxants may also be used for short-term relief of muscle spasms. Opioids are generally reserved for severe pain and are used with caution due to the risk of dependence and side effects.

Manual Therapy

Manual therapy, including spinal manipulation and mobilization, is another non-invasive treatment option. It is often used in conjunction with exercise or physical therapy. Evidence suggests that spinal manipulation can be moderately effective for acute LBP and may reduce the need for pain medications (Paige et al., 2017).

Psychological Interventions

Cognitive-behavioral therapy (CBT) has proven effective, especially in patients with chronic or recurrent LBP. Psychological interventions address the emotional and behavioral aspects of pain and can improve coping strategies, reduce fear-avoidance beliefs, and enhance patient engagement in physical activities (Kamper et al., 2015).

Interventional Treatments

For patients who do not respond to conservative treatments, interventional procedures may be considered. Epidural steroid injections are often used for radicular pain caused by nerve root compression. While these injections may provide short-term relief, their long-term benefits are uncertain (Chou et al., 2015). Other options include facet joint injections, radiofrequency ablation, and intradiscal therapies.

Surgical Interventions

Surgical treatment is typically reserved for patients with structural abnormalities (e.g., herniated discs, spinal stenosis) who do not improve with conservative care. Common surgical procedures include discectomy, laminectomy, and spinal fusion. While surgery can offer significant relief for select patients, it carries risks and should be considered only after a thorough evaluation (Deyo et al., 2010).

Multidisciplinary and Integrated Approaches

The most effective management of chronic LBP often involves a multidisciplinary approach that includes physicians, physical therapists, psychologists, and other healthcare providers. Integrative medicine techniques such as acupuncture, yoga, and mindfulness-based stress reduction have shown promising results for some individuals (Cherkin et al., 2016).

Conclusion

Effective treatment of low back pain is not a one-size-fits-all endeavor. The optimal approach depends on the nature and cause of the pain, as well as individual patient factors. Non-invasive, conservative therapies are the foundation of treatment, with interventional and surgical options reserved for more severe or refractory cases. A patient-centered, evidence-based, and multidisciplinary strategy is essential for improving outcomes and quality of life in individuals with low back pain.

Chapter 10
Support (Mental Health)

Low back pain (LBP) is one of the most common musculoskeletal disorders worldwide, affecting approximately 80% of adults at some point in their lives (Hoy et al., 2014). While much of the focus in treatment has been placed on physical and medical interventions, there is growing recognition of the essential role mental health and psychosocial support play in managing and recovering from LBP. Chronic pain not only impacts the body but also the mind, often resulting in depression, anxiety, fear-avoidance behaviors, and social isolation. Mental support strategies, including cognitive-behavioral therapy (CBT), mindfulness, education, and social support, have been shown to significantly improve outcomes in individuals suffering from LBP (Nicholas et al., 2011).

The Psychological Impact of Low Back Pain

The experience of chronic low back pain often leads to a cycle of psychological distress. Depression and anxiety are common comorbidities that exacerbate pain perception and reduce engagement in physical therapy or activity (Bair et al., 2003). Fear-avoidance beliefs—the idea that movement will worsen the pain—can lead to reduced mobility and deconditioning, further compounding the issue (Vlaeyen & Linton, 2000). These psychological consequences underscore the need for comprehensive mental health support in LBP management plans.

Cognitive-Behavioral Therapy (CBT)

CBT is among the most effective psychological interventions for managing chronic LBP. It works by helping patients reframe negative thoughts, develop coping skills, and engage in gradual activity resumption. Several randomized controlled trials have demonstrated that CBT can reduce pain-related disability, decrease emotional distress, and improve quality of life in individuals with chronic LBP (Morley et al., 1999; Hoffman et al., 2007).

Mindfulness and Meditation

Mindfulness-based stress reduction (MBSR) programs have shown promising results for chronic pain, including LBP. Mindfulness helps individuals cultivate awareness of bodily sensations and emotions without judgment, thereby reducing the emotional reactivity to pain (Kabat-Zinn, 1982). Studies have found that participants in mindfulness interventions experience improved pain acceptance and reduced pain intensity (Cherkin et al., 2016).

Psychoeducation and Patient Empowerment

Education plays a crucial role in mitigating fear and misconceptions about LBP. Empowering patients with knowledge about pain physiology, self-management techniques, and realistic recovery expectations can significantly reduce anxiety and promote active participation in rehabilitation (Louw et al., 2011). Pain neuroscience education (PNE), in particular, has emerged as an effective approach to help patients understand that chronic pain does not always signify ongoing injury.

Social and Peer Support

Chronic LBP can lead to social withdrawal, creating a sense of isolation. Peer support groups and family involvement have shown to enhance emotional well-being and encourage adherence to treatment plans. Support systems provide validation, reduce stigma, and can positively affect motivation and outlook (Martinez-Calderon et al., 2018). Involving family members in therapy also helps build a supportive home environment that fosters recovery.

Integrative Mental Health Approaches

Interdisciplinary pain management programs that include psychologists, physical therapists, and physicians provide a holistic approach to treating LBP. These programs combine physical rehabilitation with psychological interventions, offering individualized care that addresses both the mind and the body. Evidence suggests that such integrated care leads to better functional and psychosocial outcomes than single-modality treatment (Kamper et al., 2015).

Conclusion

Mental support is an essential, yet often underutilized, component in the treatment of low back pain. Addressing the psychological and emotional dimensions of pain not only improves mental health outcomes but also enhances physical recovery. Clinicians should adopt a biopsychosocial model when managing LBP and ensure access to mental health resources such as CBT, mindfulness, education, and peer support. With comprehensive care, patients are more likely to achieve long-term relief and an improved quality of life.

Chapter 11
Low Back Exercises for Low Back Pain

Understanding the Role of Exercise in LBP Management

Exercise is essential in restoring mobility, strengthening supporting musculature, and promoting spinal stability. It also helps in reducing fear-avoidance behaviors and improving functional outcomes (Shamsi et al., 2015). Unlike passive modalities, exercise encourages active patient involvement, which is critical for long-term management.

There are several forms of exercise used to manage LBP, including stretching, strengthening, stabilization, aerobic conditioning, and functional movement training. Each type targets specific deficits commonly seen in individuals with LBP.

Stretching Exercises

Stretching exercises aim to improve flexibility of the lumbar spine, pelvis, and lower extremity muscles, particularly the hamstrings, hip flexors, and erector spinae. Tightness in these muscles can alter biomechanics and increase strain on the lumbar spine (McGill, 2016).

Examples:

- Knee-to-chest stretch
- Cat-cow stretch
- Lumbar rotation stretches

Stretching should be done daily and maintained for at least 20–30 seconds per stretch to achieve flexibility gains.

Strengthening Exercises

Strengthening the core musculature is critical to supporting the spine and reducing LBP. Key muscles include the transverse abdominis, multifidus, gluteals, and paraspinal muscles. Weakness in these areas is frequently associated with poor lumbar spine control (Hodges & Richardson, 1996).

Examples:

- Bridges
- Bird-dogs
- Planks
- Pelvic tilts

Strengthening exercises should be performed 2–3 times per week and progressively increased in resistance or duration as tolerated.

Stabilization Exercises

Spinal stabilization exercises focus on maintaining neutral spine positioning during dynamic movements. These exercises improve motor control and reduce the risk of reinjury (Akuthota & Nadler, 2004).

Examples:

- Abdominal bracing
- Quadruped arm/leg raises
- Side planks
- Swiss ball exercises

Emphasis is placed on slow, controlled movements with attention to proper alignment and core engagement.

Aerobic Conditioning

Aerobic exercises such as walking, swimming, or biking are beneficial for overall conditioning and help maintain body weight, which reduces stress on the lumbar spine (Searle et al., 2015). Aerobic activity also increases blood flow and promotes healing in soft tissues.

It is recommended that patients with LBP engage in moderate aerobic activity for at least 30 minutes on most days of the week, depending on tolerance.

Functional Movement Training

This approach involves training patients to move efficiently during everyday activities such as bending, lifting, and sitting. Teaching body mechanics and ergonomics is crucial to prevent further injury.

Examples:

- Hip hinge training
- Squatting techniques
- Safe lifting practices

Implementation and Safety Considerations

Before initiating any exercise program, a thorough physical assessment should be performed. Exercises should be individualized based on pain severity, functional limitations, and comorbidities. Patients should be educated to avoid movements that exacerbate pain and to progress exercises gradually.

Supervised physical therapy is often beneficial, especially in the early stages. Over time, patients should transition to an independent home-based program.

Conclusion

Exercise therapy is a foundational component of effective LBP management. When properly prescribed, exercises improve mobility, strength, and stability, ultimately reducing pain and improving quality of life. Integrating different exercise modalities tailored to patient needs yields the best outcomes. Continued patient education and engagement are essential for long-term success in managing low back pain through exercise.

Chapter 12
Finding the Right Doctor

Low back pain (LBP) is among the most prevalent musculoskeletal disorders worldwide, affecting nearly 80% of people at some point in their lives (Maher et al., 2017). When back pain persists or intensifies, selecting the right healthcare provider becomes crucial for accurate diagnosis, effective treatment, and long-term recovery. This chapter discusses the types of medical professionals who treat low back pain, the steps involved in selecting the right doctor, and key considerations such as credentials, communication style, and treatment approach.

Understanding the Spectrum of Low Back Pain Care

LBP is complex, often resulting from a combination of mechanical, neurological, and psychosocial factors (Hartvigsen et al., 2018). Consequently, care for LBP spans several medical disciplines. Understanding the roles of different practitioners can help patients make informed decisions.

1. Primary Care Providers (PCPs)

PCPs, including family physicians and internists, are usually the first point of contact. They provide initial evaluations, order imaging, if necessary, prescribe medications, and refer patients to specialists when needed.

2. Chiropractors

Chiropractors focus on spinal manipulation and physical adjustments. They may be suitable for managing mechanical LBP, particularly when no red flags—such as infection or neurological symptoms—are present.

3. Physical Therapists

Physical therapists (PTs) specialize in movement and function. They design exercise regimens to improve mobility, strength, and posture, and they provide manual therapy for pain relief and rehabilitation.

4. Orthopedic Surgeons and Neurosurgeons

When conservative treatments fail, or when pain results from structural abnormalities such as herniated discs, surgeons may be consulted. However, surgery is typically considered only after other treatments have been exhausted (Deyo et al., 2010).

5. Pain Management Specialists

These physicians, often trained in anesthesiology or physiatry, offer interventions such as injections, nerve blocks, or implantable devices to manage chronic pain.

6. Rheumatologists

For patients whose LBP may stem from inflammatory or autoimmune conditions (e.g., ankylosing spondylitis), rheumatologists provide specialized care and diagnostic expertise.

How to Find the Right Doctor

1. Identify Your Needs

The type and duration of your pain, as well as any prior treatments, should guide your choice. Acute, uncomplicated LBP may be addressed by a PCP or PT, while chronic or severe cases may warrant a multidisciplinary team.

2. Verify Credentials

Board certification, state licensure, and specialization are basic credentials to verify. Look for providers with experience specifically in spine or musculoskeletal care.

3. Check Experience and Reviews

Online platforms can provide patient reviews and treatment outcomes. However, reviews should be interpreted carefully and used in conjunction with professional qualifications.

4. Consultation and Communication

The initial consultation is a critical step. The right doctor will take a thorough history, listen to your concerns, explain options clearly, and respect your preferences.

5. Evaluate Treatment Philosophy

Different providers may have varying approaches—some may favor medication, others physical therapy, and some may integrate alternative treatments. Seek a provider whose approach aligns with evidence-based guidelines and your personal values.

Red Flags and When to Seek Immediate Care

While most back pain is benign, certain symptoms warrant urgent attention. These include:

- Loss of bladder or bowel control
- Severe or progressive neurological deficits
- History of trauma, cancer, or systemic illness

If such symptoms are present, immediate consultation with a physician, preferably in an emergency setting—is essential.

The Value of a Multidisciplinary Approach

Evidence supports the benefit of multidisciplinary care in treating complex or chronic LBP (Kamper et al., 2015). Integrating physical therapy, psychological support, medication management, and patient education offers a holistic approach that often results in better outcomes.

Conclusion

Finding the right doctor for low back pain is a personal, often trial-and-error process, but it is foundational to effective care and recovery. Understanding the types of providers available, their qualifications, and their treatment approaches can empower patients to make informed choices. Collaboration, communication, and shared decision-making remain at the heart of high-quality, patient-centered care.

Chapter 13
A Medical Second Opinion

Low back pain (LBP) is a leading cause of disability worldwide, affecting people of all ages and contributing significantly to healthcare utilization and economic burden (Wu et al., 2020). Due to its multifactorial etiology and the broad spectrum of treatment options—from conservative care to invasive procedures—patients with LBP often face complex decisions regarding their diagnosis and treatment plan. In such scenarios, seeking a medical second opinion can be a valuable tool to ensure accurate diagnosis, explore alternative treatments, and avoid unnecessary procedures.

The Role of Second Opinions in Low Back Pain Management

Second medical opinions provide patients with an opportunity to verify or challenge the initial diagnosis and treatment recommendation. In the context of LBP, where clinical presentations can be ambiguous and management strategies vary widely, second opinions offer clarity and confidence. Research shows that second opinions frequently lead to changes in diagnosis or treatment, especially in cases involving recommendations for surgery or advanced imaging (Orenstein et al., 2020).

Patients are particularly encouraged to seek second opinions when faced with recommendations for spinal surgery, long-term opioid use, or costly diagnostic interventions. Such decisions have profound implications for quality of life, cost, and long-term outcomes. A second opinion can help avoid overtreatment, identify less invasive options, or confirm the appropriateness of the original recommendation (Gronlund et al., 2021).

Common Scenarios Warranting a Second Opinion

There are several clinical scenarios in which a second opinion should be considered in LBP cases:

- Surgical Recommendations: If spinal surgery is advised, a second opinion can assess whether conservative options have been exhausted or if the surgery is indeed the most appropriate path (Deyo et al., 2015).
- Inconclusive Diagnosis: When diagnostic tests yield unclear or conflicting results, a fresh perspective may uncover overlooked causes or alternative interpretations.
- Persistent or Worsening Symptoms: If symptoms persist despite treatment, a second opinion may suggest new diagnostic avenues or identify gaps in the treatment strategy.
- Patient Doubts: Patients who feel uncomfortable or uncertain about their care plan should be encouraged to seek another expert's assessment.

Benefits of a Second Opinion

The potential benefits of a second opinion for LBP include:

- Improved Diagnostic Accuracy: An additional review of imaging, physical exams, and clinical history can lead to more precise diagnosis.
- Treatment Optimization: Patients may be presented with less invasive or more cost-effective treatment alternatives.
- Increased Patient Confidence: Knowing that multiple experts agree on a treatment plan enhances trust and compliance.
- Avoidance of Unnecessary Procedures: Second opinions can prevent patients from undergoing surgeries or interventions that may offer limited benefit.

A study by Lentz et al. (2022) found that second opinions for spinal conditions led to changes in treatment in nearly 45% of cases, highlighting the critical role these consultations can play in improving patient outcomes.

Challenges and Considerations

While beneficial, obtaining a second opinion may not always be straightforward. Barriers can include limited access to specialists, insurance restrictions, logistical delays, and patient hesitation. Furthermore, differing opinions among healthcare providers can create confusion, requiring clear communication and guidance to help patients make informed decisions.

Healthcare providers can support patients by encouraging open dialogue and referring them to qualified specialists who can offer a balanced second opinion. Institutions with multidisciplinary spine centers may offer coordinated second opinion services, combining perspectives from orthopedic, neurology, physical therapy, and pain management specialists.

Conclusion

Medical second opinions represent a valuable tool in the management of low back pain, especially given the diagnostic complexity and treatment variability associated with this condition. By providing an additional layer of evaluation, second opinions help patients make informed, confident, and personalized decisions regarding their care. As healthcare moves toward more patient-centered models, promoting access to second opinions is essential in improving quality of care and optimizing outcomes for individuals suffering from low back pain.

Chapter 14
Hospitals for Surgery - The last Resort

Low back pain (LBP) is a common and often debilitating condition, affecting millions of individuals globally. In most cases, it is managed with conservative treatment options, including physical therapy, medications, and lifestyle modifications. However, for a small subset of patients who experience persistent pain and functional limitations despite exhaustive non-surgical interventions, low back surgery becomes the last resort. Choosing the right hospital for such a critical intervention is paramount. This chapter explores when surgery is appropriate, the types of surgical options available, the qualities of hospitals that offer top-tier spine care, and what patients should consider when surgery is inevitable.

When Surgery Becomes Necessary

Surgical intervention for low back pain is typically reserved for cases involving structural issues that have not responded to conservative treatment. Indications for surgery include:

- Herniated discs causing severe nerve compression
- Spinal stenosis
- Spondylolisthesis
- Severe degenerative disc disease
- Spinal deformities (e.g., scoliosis)
- Trauma or tumor-related instability (Chou et al., 2009)

Surgery is generally considered only after 6–12 months of failed conservative care unless there is neurological impairment or an emergent issue such as cauda equina syndrome (Deyo et al., 2010).

Types of Low Back Surgery

Common surgical procedures include:

- Discectomy: Removal of herniated disc material
- Laminectomy: Removal of part of the vertebral bone to relieve pressure
- Spinal fusion: Joining two or more vertebrae to stabilize the spine
- Artificial disc replacement: Insertion of a prosthetic disc to maintain motion

Minimally invasive techniques have become more prevalent and are associated with quicker recovery times and reduced postoperative complications (Wang et al., 2021).

Selecting the Right Hospital

When surgery is the last resort, choosing a hospital with a comprehensive spine program is essential. Top hospitals often offer:

1. Multidisciplinary Spine Teams
Hospitals with integrated teams of orthopedic surgeons, neurosurgeons, physiatrists, and pain specialists offer collaborative care and better outcomes.

2. Advanced Diagnostic and Surgical Technology
High-performing hospitals utilize intraoperative imaging, robotic-assisted surgery, and computer navigation for precision and safety.

3. High Surgical Volumes
Facilities performing a higher number of spine surgeries tend to have better outcomes and fewer complications (Farrokhi et al., 2017).

4. Postoperative Rehabilitation Programs
Comprehensive recovery plans including physical therapy and pain management are crucial for successful outcomes.

5. Patient Satisfaction and Outcome Tracking
Hospitals that track patient-reported outcomes and surgical success rates provide transparency and continuous quality improvement.

Leading Hospitals for Low Back Surgery

According to U.S. News & World Report and other medical rankings, the following hospitals are consistently recognized for excellence in spine surgery:

- Mayo Clinic (Rochester, MN)
- Cleveland Clinic (Cleveland, OH)
- Hospital for Special Surgery (New York, NY)
- Johns Hopkins Hospital (Baltimore, MD)
- Cedars-Sinai Medical Center (Los Angeles, CA)

These institutions offer world-class care, cutting-edge surgical techniques, and integrated recovery programs that are critical when surgery becomes the final option.

Risks and Expectations

Despite advances, spine surgery carries risks including infection, nerve damage, and failure to relieve pain. Informed consent and clear communication with the surgical team are essential. Success rates vary depending on the procedure and patient condition. Generally, outcomes improve significantly with proper patient selection and hospital quality (Andrade et al., 2015).

Conclusion

Low back surgery should always be considered a last resort after all non-surgical options have been exhausted. For those requiring surgery, selecting the right hospital is critical to maximizing outcomes and minimizing complications. Hospitals with high surgical volumes, experienced multidisciplinary teams, and strong rehabilitation programs are best equipped to handle these complex cases. Making an informed choice can lead to a significant improvement in pain and quality of life for those who undergo spinal surgery.

Chapter 15

Medicines for Low Back Pain

Low back pain (LBP) is a leading cause of disability globally, affecting individuals across all age groups. It often interferes with daily activities and contributes to significant healthcare expenditures. While non-pharmacologic therapies such as exercise and physical therapy are first-line interventions, medications play a critical role in managing pain and enhancing function, particularly during acute or severe episodes (Qaseem et al., 2017). This chapter explores various classes of medications used for low back pain, their mechanisms of action, clinical effectiveness, side effects, and appropriate usage guidelines.

1. Nonsteroidal Anti-Inflammatory Drugs (NSAIDs)

NSAIDs are considered first-line pharmacologic treatment for both acute and chronic LBP due to their anti-inflammatory and analgesic effects. Common NSAIDs include ibuprofen, naproxen, and diclofenac. They work by inhibiting cyclooxygenase (COX) enzymes, which reduces prostaglandin synthesis and alleviates inflammation and pain (Deyo et al., 2015). Despite their effectiveness, NSAIDs carry risks such as gastrointestinal bleeding, renal dysfunction, and cardiovascular events, particularly with long-term use.

2. Acetaminophen (Paracetamol)

Acetaminophen is often used for mild to moderate pain but has fallen out of favor for LBP due to limited efficacy. According to a large randomized trial, acetaminophen was found to be no more effective than placebo in reducing pain intensity or improving function in patients with acute LBP (Williams et al., 2014). However, it may still be appropriate for individuals who cannot tolerate NSAIDs.

3. Muscle Relaxants

Muscle relaxants, including cyclobenzaprine, tizanidine, and methocarbamol, are frequently prescribed for acute LBP associated with muscle spasms. These medications may offer short-term pain relief but are associated with sedation, dizziness, and potential for dependency (Furlan et al., 2003). They should be used cautiously and for limited durations.

4. Opioids

Opioids such as tramadol, hydrocodone, and oxycodone are sometimes used for severe LBP unresponsive to other treatments. While effective for short-term relief, opioids are not recommended for long-term management due to high risks of tolerance, dependence, overdose, and addiction (Chou et al., 2007). Guidelines recommend reserving opioids for select cases and using the lowest effective dose for the shortest duration.

5. Antidepressants

Tricyclic antidepressants (e.g., amitriptyline) and serotonin-norepinephrine reuptake inhibitors (e.g., duloxetine) may be beneficial for chronic LBP, especially when there is a coexisting mood disorder or neuropathic pain component. These medications influence central pain pathways and can improve both pain and quality of life (Krebs et al., 2018). Common side effects include dry mouth, drowsiness, and weight gain.

6. Anticonvulsants

Gabapentin and pregabalin, commonly used for neuropathic pain, are sometimes prescribed for chronic LBP with radiating leg pain or sciatica. However, evidence of their effectiveness for nonspecific LBP is limited, and they can cause side effects such as dizziness and fatigue (Enke et al., 2018). They should not be used routinely unless there is a clear neuropathic component.

7. Topical Agents

Topical NSAIDs and lidocaine patches offer localized pain relief with fewer systemic effects. These are particularly useful in older adults or those at risk of systemic medication side effects. They are most effective for mild to moderate localized pain (Gatti et al., 2016).

8. Emerging Therapies

Research is ongoing into alternative pharmacologic options, such as cannabinoid-based treatments and biologics targeting inflammatory pathways. However, current evidence is insufficient to support their routine use for LBP (Ablin et al., 2016).

Conclusion

Medications for low back pain can play a valuable role in reducing discomfort and enhancing function, especially in the acute phase or in cases of moderate to severe pain. However, they must be used judiciously, with careful consideration of the patient's individual risk factors and in combination with non-pharmacologic approaches. Clinical guidelines emphasize starting with the least invasive options and tailoring treatment plans to minimize long-term medication dependence.

<u>Disclaimer:</u>

This book is for reference only. It is not to suggest, recommend or condone any medical advice. For specific medical assistance please reach out to a licensed medical professional. Everyone has a different and unique journey, and this book only covers mine.

Chapter 16

Difficulty in the Reliability of the Medical field

Low back pain (LBP) remains one of the most common reasons for seeking medical care, yet there is significant difficulty in establishing reliable diagnosis, treatment, and prognosis pathways. The complexity of the human spine, combined with the multifactorial origins of back pain, has led to variability in medical opinion, diagnostic accuracy, and treatment outcomes. These inconsistencies raise questions about the reliability of the medical system in effectively managing LBP. This chapter explores the key areas where reliability is compromised and discusses potential solutions to enhance consistency and trust in the care of patients with LBP.

Diagnostic Variability

One major challenge in the medical field's reliability regarding LBP is the inconsistency in diagnostic practices. Despite the widespread use of imaging modalities such as MRI and CT scans, studies have shown that these tools often fail to correlate with symptoms (Jensen et al., 1994). Many patients present with significant pain despite normal imaging, while others show abnormal imaging findings without clinical symptoms. This discrepancy undermines confidence in diagnostics and can lead to both over-treatment and under-treatment.

Furthermore, physical examinations are subject to significant variability among providers. Clinicians differ in their interpretations of tests like straight leg raises, range of motion assessments, and neurological evaluations. This lack of standardization contributes to inconsistent diagnoses and patient confusion (Deyo & Weinstein, 2001).

Treatment Inconsistencies

Treatment plans for LBP vary widely among practitioners, often reflecting personal preference more than evidence-based practice. For example, one physician may prescribe opioids, another may recommend physical therapy, and a third may suggest surgery for the same patient scenario. This variability can lead to conflicting advice, fragmented care, and patient dissatisfaction (Chou et al., 2007).

Moreover, some treatments lack long-term efficacy. Surgical interventions, such as spinal fusion, are frequently performed despite limited evidence supporting their superiority over conservative management (Fritzell et al., 2001). This adds to the perception that the medical system lacks a reliable and consistent approach to managing LBP.

Bias and Overmedicalization

Another barrier to reliability is the presence of bias in clinical decision-making. Patients with similar symptoms may receive different treatments based on age, gender, socioeconomic status, or even the provider's specialty. Specialists may recommend interventions aligned with their training rather than the patient's best interests, a phenomenon known as the "treatment bias" (Deyo, 2002).

In addition, the healthcare system often promotes overmedicalization of LBP. The use of unnecessary imaging, invasive procedures, and prolonged pharmacologic therapies not only fails to improve outcomes but also increases costs and exposes patients to avoidable risks (Walker et al., 2003).

Patient Experience and Trust

The inconsistencies in diagnosis and treatment negatively affect patient trust in the healthcare system. Patients frequently report feeling dismissed or confused due to contradictory opinions. Chronic LBP patients, in particular, may undergo multiple consultations with varying explanations and treatment suggestions, leading to frustration and decreased adherence to care plans (Synnott et al., 2015).

This erosion of trust has downstream effects, including increased reliance on alternative therapies, non-compliance with medical advice, and exacerbation of psychological comorbidities such as anxiety and depression.

Improving Reliability in LBP Management

To address these challenges, the medical field must focus on evidence-based guidelines, interdisciplinary collaboration, and shared decision-making. Standardized clinical pathways, like those promoted by the American College of Physicians, can help reduce unwarranted variation (Qaseem et al., 2017). Greater use of multidisciplinary teams—combining primary care, physical therapy, pain management, and mental health services—can offer more holistic and consistent care.

Additionally, increased emphasis on patient education and involvement in treatment decisions may improve satisfaction and outcomes. Clear communication about diagnostic uncertainty, treatment options, and expected outcomes foster trust and shared responsibility.

Conclusion

Low back pain exemplifies the difficulty in ensuring reliability within the medical field. The variability in diagnostic accuracy, treatment practices, and patient-provider communication reflects a fragmented system that often fails to meet patient expectations. By recognizing and addressing these gaps, the medical community can work toward a more consistent, evidence-based, and patient-centered approach to LBP care.

Chapter 17
Physical Therapy

Low back pain (LBP) is one of the most prevalent and disabling musculoskeletal conditions globally, with profound personal and socioeconomic consequences. It affects individuals of all ages and is a leading cause of work absenteeism and healthcare utilization (Hartvigsen et al., 2018). While pharmacological and surgical interventions have roles in management, physical therapy has emerged as a cornerstone in both acute and chronic LBP care. Physical therapy aims to reduce pain, restore function, and prevent recurrence through evidence-based exercise programs, manual therapy, education, and lifestyle modifications.

Understanding Low Back Pain

LBP is broadly classified into three categories: acute (lasting less than six weeks), subacute (6–12 weeks), and chronic (more than 12 weeks) (Qaseem et al., 2017). Most cases are nonspecific, meaning there is no identifiable anatomical cause, such as a herniated disc or spinal stenosis. Due to this complexity, a biopsychosocial approach is advocated, and physical therapists are well-positioned to deliver such holistic care.

Goals of Physical Therapy in LBP

The overarching goals of physical therapy for LBP are:

1. Pain Reduction: Through modalities such as manual therapy, therapeutic ultrasound, or electrical stimulation.
2. Restoration of Mobility and Strength: Targeted exercises improve muscle imbalances and postural issues.
3. Functional Rehabilitation: Return to work, sports, or daily activities is facilitated through progressive functional training.
4. Patient Education: Teaching patients self-management strategies and addressing fear-avoidance beliefs helps prevent chronicity.

Exercise Therapy

Exercise is the most consistently recommended intervention for LBP. Types of exercises include:

- Stretching and Flexibility Training: Targets tight musculature (e.g., hamstrings, hip flexors).
- Strengthening Exercises: Focuses on core stability (e.g., transversus abdominis, multifidus muscles).
- Aerobic Conditioning: Improves general health and reduces pain perception.
- Motor Control Exercises: Re-educate muscle activation patterns to support spinal structures.

Research indicates that tailored exercise programs are more effective than passive treatments and general exercise alone (Searle et al., 2015).

Manual Therapy

Manual therapy techniques such as spinal manipulation and mobilization can provide short-term pain relief, especially in acute LBP. These techniques are often combined with exercise and have shown favorable outcomes in randomized controlled trials (Delitto et al., 2012).

Education and Behavioral Strategies

Patient education is central to therapy. Key messages include:

- Pain does not always mean damage.
- Staying active is better than bed rest.
- Self-management can reduce long-term disability.

Cognitive-behavioral therapy techniques, integrated by physical therapists, have also shown benefits in chronic LBP (Nicholas et al., 2011).

Emerging Approaches and Technologies

New approaches include:

• Tele-rehabilitation: Remote delivery of therapy via video calls, which has become more prominent post-COVID-19.
• Virtual Reality (VR): Enhances patient engagement in exercise.
• Wearable Technology: Provides real-time feedback on posture and movement.

These innovations promise greater accessibility and adherence to therapy protocols.

Barriers to Physical Therapy Utilization

Despite its effectiveness, barriers include:

• Limited insurance coverage.
• Lack of awareness among patients and referring providers.
• Geographic and transportation constraints.

Efforts to promote early referral to physical therapy are essential to reduce reliance on opioids and prevent chronic disability.

Conclusion

Physical therapy is a critical, evidence-based component in the management of low back pain. Through a combination of exercise, manual therapy, education, and behavioral interventions, physical therapy not only addresses pain but also empowers individuals to take control of their health. As healthcare moves toward value-based care, integrating physical therapy early in the LBP care pathway can enhance outcomes and reduce costs.

Chapter 18
Pain Management

Low back pain (LBP) is a leading cause of disability worldwide, affecting up to 80% of individuals at some point in their lives (Hoy et al., 2014). Effective pain management is essential for improving function and quality of life in patients with both acute and chronic LBP. Management strategies often involve a multidisciplinary approach, including pharmacological treatments, specialist doctors, and a variety of medical procedures. This chapter explores the landscape of pain management for low back pain, focusing on medications, healthcare providers, and procedural interventions.

Pharmacological Management of Low Back Pain

Pharmacotherapy remains a cornerstone in the management of LBP. Medications are tailored according to the severity, duration, and underlying cause of pain.

Non-Opioid Analgesics

Non-steroidal anti-inflammatory drugs (NSAIDs) such as ibuprofen and naproxen are often the first line of treatment for acute LBP due to their efficacy in reducing inflammation and pain (van Tulder et al., 2000). Acetaminophen is also commonly used, although recent studies suggest it may be less effective for LBP than previously believed (Williams et al., 2014).

Muscle Relaxants and Anticonvulsants

For patients with muscle spasms or neuropathic components of pain, muscle relaxants such as cyclobenzaprine and anticonvulsants like gabapentin can be beneficial (Chou et al., 2017). These drugs target different pain pathways, contributing to multi-modal pain control.

Opioids

Opioids are reserved for severe pain that is unresponsive to other treatments due to the risk of dependence and side effects. Guidelines recommend cautious use with close monitoring, especially in chronic cases (Dowell et al., 2016).

Pain Management Specialists

Effective LBP management often involves collaboration among various healthcare providers.

Primary Care Physicians

Primary care doctors are typically the first point of contact for patients with LBP. They assess, diagnose, initiate first-line treatments, and refer patients to specialists as needed.

Pain Management Specialists

These are physicians with advanced training in diagnosing and treating chronic pain, typically from backgrounds in anesthesiology, neurology, or physical medicine and rehabilitation. They use a combination of medications, interventional techniques, and referrals to physical or psychological therapy (Manchikanti et al., 2009).

Neurologists and Orthopedic Surgeons

Neurologists may be involved when neurological symptoms like sciatica are present, while orthopedic surgeons handle structural issues of the spine. Surgical intervention is considered a last resort after conservative treatments fail (Deyo et al., 2010).

Interventional Pain Management Procedures

A variety of procedures may be used to manage persistent LBP.

Epidural Steroid Injections

These injections are often used to reduce inflammation and pain in patients with disc herniation or spinal stenosis. While they offer short-term relief, their long-term benefits are still debated (Chou et al., 2015).

Facet Joint Injections and Medial Branch Blocks

Facet joints can be a source of chronic LBP. Targeted injections or nerve blocks help diagnose and treat this pain source effectively (Manchikanti et al., 2003).

Radiofrequency Ablation (RFA)

RFA uses heat to destroy nerve fibers carrying pain signals. It is often employed after successful diagnostic blocks and provides relief for several months (Cohen et al., 2008).

Spinal Cord Stimulation

For intractable pain, especially when neuropathic in nature, spinal cord stimulation may be considered. This involves implanting a device that modifies pain signals before they reach the brain (Kumar et al., 2007).

Conclusion

Managing low back pain effectively requires a multifaceted approach combining pharmacologic treatments, professional guidance from specialized doctors, and sometimes interventional procedures. Understanding the appropriate use of each modality is crucial to minimizing pain, restoring function, and improving quality of life for patients.

Chapter 19
Epidurals, Avoiding Additional Surgery

Low back pain (LBP) is one of the leading causes of disability worldwide and represents a significant public health burden. While surgery may be indicated in certain severe or progressive cases, many patients experience recurrent symptoms even after surgical intervention. In such cases, the pursuit of additional surgery is not always ideal due to risks, cost, and inconsistent outcomes. Epidural steroid injections (ESIs), a minimally invasive procedure, offer a non-surgical alternative to manage pain and inflammation, often allowing patients to avoid further surgical intervention. This chapter explores the role of epidural injections in post-surgical pain management, their mechanisms of action, efficacy, and place in the continuum of care for patients with persistent or recurrent low back pain.

Understanding Epidural Injections

Epidural steroid injections involve the administration of corticosteroids and sometimes anesthetics into the epidural space of the spinal column. This space surrounds the dural sac, which encases the spinal cord and nerve roots. The objective is to reduce inflammation and alleviate pain caused by nerve root irritation or compression, commonly resulting from herniated discs, spinal stenosis, or failed back surgery syndrome (FBSS) (Manchikanti et al., 2013).

Three primary approaches are used for epidural injection:

1. Interlaminar – through the midline between the vertebrae.
2. Transforaminal – directed into the foramen, the exit point of the nerve root.
3. Caudal – through the sacral hiatus at the base of the spine.

Each approach has its indications and efficacy profile depending on the patient's specific pathology and surgical history (Benzon et al., 2015).

The Challenge of Failed Back Surgery Syndrome

Failed back surgery syndrome, also known as post-laminectomy syndrome, describes chronic pain following spinal surgery, often without a clear anatomical cause. FBSS is notoriously difficult to treat, and additional surgeries frequently have diminishing returns (Chan & Peng, 2011). Reoperation rates vary, with some studies indicating up to 20% of patients undergoing repeat procedures (Deyo et al., 2011). Epidural injections provide a critical intervention point in these cases, particularly when diagnostic imaging and clinical symptoms suggest nerve inflammation without structural instability.

Mechanism of Action

The corticosteroids used in ESIs suppress the production of inflammatory mediators such as prostaglandins and leukotrienes, reduce capillary permeability, and inhibit ectopic discharges from nerve roots (Abdi et al., 2007). Anesthetic agents provide immediate pain relief and help identify the source of pain. By reducing inflammation around compressed or irritated nerve roots, ESIs can significantly decrease pain and improve function, often delaying or avoiding the need for further surgical exploration.

Efficacy and Outcomes

The literature presents mixed but generally favorable evidence for the use of ESIs, particularly in patients who have had prior back surgery. A systematic review by Manchikanti et al. (2012) found moderate evidence supporting the short- to intermediate-term effectiveness of epidural injections for radicular pain, especially when administered via the transforaminal route.

Notably, transforaminal injections are often more targeted and effective for radicular symptoms, while interlaminar and caudal injections may be preferable for diffuse or axial pain (Gajraj, 2005). Repeat injections, typically spaced weeks apart, may be necessary for sustained benefit. In some cases, these injections can provide a window for physical therapy or rehabilitation to take effect.

Risks and Considerations

While generally safe, epidural injections are not without risks. Potential complications include infection, bleeding, dural puncture, nerve damage, and, in rare cases, spinal cord infarction (Benzon et al., 2015). Additionally, the systemic effects of corticosteroids—such as elevated blood glucose and suppressed immunity—should be considered, especially in patients with diabetes or chronic illness.

Appropriate patient selection, image-guided techniques (usually with fluoroscopy or CT), and adherence to sterile procedures significantly reduce these risks.

When Epidurals Help Avoid Additional Surgery

Epidural injections are most effective in patients with:

- Recurrent radiculopathy after surgery,
- MRI-confirmed inflammation or disc pathology without mechanical instability,
- Contraindications to surgery,
- A desire to avoid repeat surgery due to age, comorbidities, or personal preference.

In multidisciplinary pain management strategies, ESIs can reduce reliance on opioids, support rehabilitation efforts, and serve as a bridge to other therapies (Benyamin et al., 2012).

Conclusion

Epidural steroid injections are a valuable tool in the management of chronic and recurrent low back pain, particularly following surgical interventions. When used appropriately, they can reduce pain, enhance function, and help patients avoid additional surgeries. For patients with persistent pain, especially in the setting of failed back surgery syndrome, epidurals offer a less invasive, cost-effective option that complements a broader multimodal treatment approach.

Chapter 20
Losing hope through failed surgeries

Low back pain (LBP) is one of the most prevalent causes of disability worldwide and leads millions to seek relief through surgical intervention. While surgery may provide significant relief for some, for others, the journey is marred by persistent or worsened pain, complications, and emotional exhaustion. This chapter explores the devastating psychological and emotional consequences of failed low back pain surgeries, the clinical implications, and the need for integrative, patient-centered approaches in addressing failed back surgery syndrome (FBSS).

Understanding Failed Back Surgery Syndrome

Failed back surgery syndrome (FBSS), sometimes referred to as post-laminectomy syndrome, describes a condition in which patients experience persistent or recurrent pain following spinal surgery. It is estimated that up to 40% of patients undergoing lumbar spine surgery may develop FBSS (Chan & Peng, 2011). Contributing factors include surgical complications, misdiagnosis of the pain source, nerve damage, scar tissue formation, or poor surgical candidacy.

FBSS is not merely a physical diagnosis—it reflects a broader collapse of patient expectations and medical trust. Patients often undergo surgery with high hopes, only to face continued pain and reduced function. This leads to cycles of disappointment, helplessness, and, ultimately, hopelessness (Buchbinder et al., 2009).

The Psychological Toll of Surgical Failure

For many patients, the road to surgery is already paved with suffering. When that journey ends in failure, the psychological burden intensifies. Depression, anxiety, post-traumatic stress symptoms, and even suicidal ideation have been reported among individuals experiencing failed surgeries (Block et al., 2001). The promise of a cure becomes a cruel deception, fostering deep mistrust of the healthcare system.

Hope plays a critical role in coping with chronic pain. When hope is lost after multiple failed interventions, patients may withdraw from rehabilitation efforts, reduce social interaction, and lose the motivation to seek alternative therapies. Studies show that chronic pain, when combined with failed interventions, exacerbates feelings of isolation and despair (Turk et al., 2011).

Impact on Quality of Life and Identity

Chronic pain is not only a physical experience but also a disruption of life roles and identity. Failed back surgeries often limit patients' ability to work, parent, socialize, or engage in previously enjoyed activities. Over time, patients may internalize a new identity centered around pain and disability, which reinforces feelings of worthlessness and hopelessness (Main et al., 2010).

Moreover, financial stress due to medical bills, lost income, and disability claims can further strain patients and their families. This multidimensional burden—physical, emotional, social, and economic—amplifies the hopelessness many feel after surgical failures.

Navigating the Aftermath: Rebuilding Hope

Despite these challenges, hope can be rekindled through comprehensive, multidisciplinary care. Pain psychology, physical therapy, non-opioid medications, neuromodulation (such as spinal cord stimulation), and cognitive-behavioral therapy (CBT) have shown promise in restoring function and improving emotional well-being after failed surgeries (Kumar et al., 2007).

Healthcare providers must take a trauma-informed, empathetic approach to these patients. Rather than viewing failed surgery as a dead end, clinicians should emphasize resilience, adapt treatment goals, and validate the patient's pain experience. Building a therapeutic alliance grounded in trust can help patients reframe their narrative from failure to adaptation and growth.

Conclusion

Failed low back pain surgeries can devastate patients' physical health and emotional spirit. When the promise of relief becomes a recurring disappointment, it erodes hope and leads to psychological and existential distress. Recognizing and addressing this hopelessness is essential. A holistic, multidisciplinary approach can offer new avenues for healing, even when surgery has failed. By prioritizing empathy and comprehensive care, healthcare providers can help patients move beyond despair and rediscover meaning and quality of life.

Chapter 21

Osteoporosis, A Potential Cause?

Low back pain (LBP) is among the most prevalent musculoskeletal complaints worldwide, affecting up to 80% of people at some point in their lives (Balagué et al., 2012). While its causes are multifactorial—ranging from muscle strain to degenerative disc disease—osteoporosis is an under-recognized but significant contributor to LBP, especially in aging populations (Sinaki, 2017). Osteoporosis is a systemic skeletal disorder characterized by reduced bone mass and microarchitectural deterioration, leading to increased bone fragility and risk of fractures (National Osteoporosis Foundation [NOF], 2023). Vertebral compression fractures, a hallmark of advanced osteoporosis, are a direct cause of acute and chronic low back pain. This chapter explores the relationship between osteoporosis and LBP, emphasizing pathophysiology, clinical presentation, diagnostic approaches, and management strategies.

Pathophysiology of Osteoporosis and Its Link to Low Back Pain

Osteoporosis develops when bone resorption outpaces bone formation, resulting in weakened bone structure (Compston et al., 2019). The vertebrae—particularly the thoracic and lumbar spine—are common sites for osteoporotic fractures due to their structural and weight-bearing roles (Fink et al., 2003). Vertebral compression fractures can occur with minimal or no trauma, causing acute pain from periosteal stretching, muscle spasm, and nerve root irritation (Gold et al., 2016).

Repeated or multiple vertebral fractures may lead to spinal deformities such as kyphosis, altering biomechanics and contributing to chronic low back pain through increased muscle fatigue, ligament strain, and abnormal load distribution (Sinaki, 2017). Additionally, these structural changes can limit mobility and impair quality of life.

Clinical Presentation and Diagnosis

Patients with osteoporotic LBP may present with sudden, severe back pain following minor movements, such as bending or lifting. Unlike muscular LBP, the pain is often localized, worse with weight bearing, and relieved by lying down (Kanis et al., 2019).

Diagnosis involves a combination of clinical assessment, imaging, and bone mineral density (BMD) measurement. Dual-energy X-ray absorptiometry (DXA) is the gold standard for assessing BMD (NOF, 2023). Spinal radiographs can reveal vertebral compression fractures, which may otherwise go undetected due to their often asymptomatic nature (Fink et al., 2003). Magnetic resonance imaging (MRI) can help differentiate acute fractures from chronic deformities and exclude other causes of back pain.

Management Strategies

Management of osteoporosis-related LBP requires a multidisciplinary approach, focusing on both fracture prevention and pain control. Pharmacologic therapy includes antiresorptive agents such as bisphosphonates or denosumab, which slow bone loss, and anabolic agents like teriparatide to stimulate bone formation (Cosman et al., 2014).

Pain management may involve analgesics, muscle relaxants, and bracing for acute fractures (Gold et al., 2016). Vertebral augmentation procedures, such as vertebroplasty or kyphoplasty, may be considered for select patients with intractable pain despite conservative measures (Clark et al., 2016).

Non-pharmacologic interventions are equally critical. Physical therapy focusing on core strengthening, posture training, and balance exercises can help maintain spinal stability and reduce the risk of falls (Sinaki, 2017). Lifestyle modifications—adequate calcium and vitamin D intake, weight-bearing exercises, and smoking cessation—are essential for long-term bone health (NOF, 2023).

Conclusion

Osteoporosis is a significant but sometimes overlooked cause of low back pain, particularly in older adults. Recognizing its role in vertebral compression fractures is crucial for timely diagnosis and management.

Addressing osteoporosis not only alleviates current pain but also reduces the risk of future fractures, spinal deformities, and related disability. Comprehensive care requires a combination of medical treatment, physical rehabilitation, and preventive strategies to optimize bone health and improve quality of life.

Chapter 22
Expenses and Consequences of Low Back Surgery

Low back pain is one of the leading causes of disability worldwide, significantly affecting quality of life and productivity (Hoy et al., 2014). When conservative treatments fail, surgery is often considered as a last resort. However, low back surgery is not only costly but also associated with a range of consequences, both expected and unforeseen. This chapter explores the financial burden, indirect costs, and physical, psychological, and social implications of low back surgery, highlighting the importance of comprehensive decision-making for patients and healthcare systems alike.

Financial Costs of Low Back Surgery

Low back surgery is among the most expensive medical interventions for musculoskeletal disorders. Direct costs include surgeon fees, hospital stays, anesthesia, postoperative care, medications, and rehabilitation services. The average cost of spinal fusion, one of the most common procedures, ranges from $50,000 to $100,000 per case in the

United States (Deyo et al., 2014). Costs vary by procedure type, hospital setting, insurance coverage, and geographic location.

In addition to upfront expenses, repeat surgeries are not uncommon. Failed Back Surgery Syndrome (FBSS) affects approximately 10–40% of patients, often leading to additional surgeries, chronic pain management, or even spinal cord stimulation, further increasing the financial burden (Thompson et al., 2021).

Indirect Costs and Economic Impact

Beyond direct medical costs, indirect costs add significant economic weight. These include lost productivity due to extended recovery times, inability to return to work, or reduced work capacity (Wong et al., 2019). Disability benefits and workers' compensation claims related to low back surgery represent substantial costs to employers and insurers.

A 2019 study estimated that the total annual indirect costs of low back pain, including surgeries, in the U.S. exceed $100 billion, primarily due to work absenteeism and reduced workforce participation (Katz, 2006; Wong et al., 2019).

Health Consequences and Risks

While many patients benefit from surgery, the risks must be carefully weighed. Complications may include infection, nerve damage, bleeding, or adverse reactions to anesthesia (Deyo et al., 2014). Some patients experience persistent or worsening pain postoperatively, leading to long-term opioid use or additional interventions.

Psychologically, failed surgical outcomes can exacerbate depression and anxiety, fueling a cycle of chronic pain and diminished hope for recovery (Thompson et al., 2021). These consequences may require further psychological and medical support, adding to the cost and complexity of care.

Social and Family Implications

The impact of surgery extends to family and social dynamics. Recovery often demands caregiver support, adjustments in daily living, and financial strain on households. Loss of income during rehabilitation can create significant stress, particularly when multiple surgeries are required.

Patients should be educated about realistic recovery expectations and supported with comprehensive care plans that address physical, mental, and social well-being (Deyo et al., 2014).

Strategies to Mitigate Costs and Risks

Given the expenses and potential consequences, careful patient selection and shared decision-making are critical. Evidence-based guidelines emphasize exhausting conservative measures—such as physical therapy, cognitive-behavioral therapy, and interventional pain management—before surgery is considered (Qaseem et al., 2017).

When surgery is indicated, multidisciplinary care, prehabilitation, and clear communication about risks and benefits can help optimize outcomes and contain costs (Wong et al., 2019).

Conclusion

Low back surgery carries significant expenses and consequences that extend beyond the operating room. Patients, families, providers, and policymakers must recognize the full scope of costs—direct, indirect, physical, psychological, and social—to make informed decisions. Future efforts should continue to refine patient selection, improve surgical techniques, and expand access to effective conservative treatments to reduce the need for surgery and its associated burdens.

Chapter 23
Exercises, Mobility, Stability and Pain Reduction

Low back pain and other musculoskeletal complaints remain leading causes of disability worldwide (Hartvigsen et al., 2018). Exercise-based interventions, when properly designed, have proven efficacy in improving mobility, enhancing stability, and reducing pain (Qaseem et al., 2017). Understanding how these elements interact is essential for clinicians, therapists, and individuals seeking to maintain function and quality of life.

The Role of Exercise in Pain Management

Exercise is a cornerstone in managing acute and chronic pain conditions. Therapeutic exercise improves blood flow, supports healing, and modulates pain perception through central and peripheral mechanisms (Geneen et al., 2017). Regular activity can reduce fear-avoidance behaviors and improve self-efficacy, both of which contribute to pain reduction (MacDonald et al., 2019).

Types of exercises often used include aerobic conditioning, strength training, flexibility training, and neuromotor exercises. Each serves a unique role in supporting mobility, stability, and overall musculoskeletal health.

Mobility: Restoring and Maintaining Range of Motion

Mobility refers to the ability of joints and muscles to move through their full functional range. Restricted mobility can lead to compensatory movement patterns, which may perpetuate pain and dysfunction (Page et al., 2012).

Stretching routines, soft tissue mobilization, and dynamic range-of-motion exercises target specific limitations. For example, lumbar and hip mobility exercises are critical for patients with low back pain to prevent compensatory overload of surrounding structures (Bishop et al., 2017).

Stability: Building Strength and Control

While mobility ensures adequate motion, stability provides the muscular control required to maintain joint integrity during movement. Poor stability can contribute to microtrauma and chronic pain (Panjabi, 1992).

Core stabilization programs, which focus on deep trunk muscles such as the transversus abdominis and multifidus, are particularly beneficial for spinal health (Hodges, 2003). Strengthening surrounding musculature, including gluteals and hip stabilizers, enhances functional control and load distribution (Akuthota & Nadler, 2004).

Integration: Combining Mobility and Stability

Optimal outcomes occur when mobility and stability exercises are combined in a functional, progressive manner. For instance, integrating dynamic movements like controlled lunges or yoga flows can simultaneously enhance flexibility and neuromuscular control (Cruz-Díaz et al., 2015).

Therapists often tailor programs to individual needs, considering factors like pain severity, movement patterns, and psychosocial influences. Consistency and gradual progression are vital to prevent flare-ups and sustain improvements.

Pain Reduction: The End Goal

Research supports that tailored exercise programs significantly reduce pain intensity and disability compared to passive treatments alone (Hayden et al., 2021). Moreover, regular exercise may have long-term protective effects against recurrent pain episodes (Shiri et al., 2018).

Mind-body practices, such as Pilates and Tai Chi, can be incorporated to address both physical and cognitive aspects of pain, offering additional benefits through relaxation and mindful movement (Hall et al., 2016).

Conclusion

A comprehensive exercise approach addressing mobility and stability is fundamental for effective pain management and prevention. Clinicians and patients alike should prioritize evidence-based, individualized programs that promote active participation and foster resilience against future pain episodes.

Chapter 24
Removal of Hardware After Lumbar Spine Surgery

Instrumented lumbar fusion is a common surgical intervention used to stabilize the spine in the treatment of degenerative conditions, deformity, trauma, or neoplasia. The use of pedicle screws, rods, interbody cages, and other fixation devices plays a pivotal role in achieving spinal stability and promoting bony fusion. While these implants are typically intended to remain in situ permanently, there are circumstances in which hardware removal becomes necessary or beneficial. This chapter reviews the indications, surgical considerations, outcomes, and complications of hardware removal in the lumbar spine, with current evidence and best practices.

Indications for Hardware Removal

Hardware removal is not routine after lumbar fusion and is typically reserved for cases where the implants are symptomatic or problematic. Common indications include:

- Persistent or new-onset pain suspected to be due to hardware irritation (e.g., muscle irritation, nerve impingement, or pseudoarthrosis)
- Infection involving the implant or surrounding tissues
- Hardware failure, including screw loosening, breakage, or migration
- Allergic or inflammatory response to implant materials
- Radiological evidence of successful fusion with ongoing mechanical symptoms

Persistent pain is one of the most frequent reasons for considering removal, particularly in cases where imaging shows adequate fusion. In such cases, patients may experience relief after hardware explantation, although outcomes can be variable (Kim et al., 2012).

Preoperative Evaluation

Prior to recommending hardware removal, a comprehensive workup is essential to determine whether symptoms are attributable to the implants.

- Radiographic assessment (plain films, CT) to evaluate the integrity of the hardware and confirm fusion
- MRI or CT myelography if neurologic symptoms are present
- Diagnostic injections, such as local anesthetic injections near the hardware, may be useful in confirming that the implants are the pain source (Yoo et al., 2008)
- Laboratory testing, including inflammatory markers (e.g., ESR, CRP), in cases of suspected infection

Decision-making must weigh the risks of reoperation against the likelihood of symptom relief. In patients with incomplete fusion (pseudoarthrosis), removal may not be advisable unless followed by revision fusion.

Surgical Technique

Hardware removal is typically performed through the original surgical approach to minimize additional soft tissue trauma. Key steps include:

1. Anesthesia: General anesthesia is administered.
2. Exposure: The original incision is reopened, and meticulous dissection is required to navigate scar tissue.
3. Removal: Screws, rods, and other components are carefully removed. Fluoroscopy may be used to localize hardware.
4. Fusion Assessment: Intraoperative assessment of fusion status is critical. If pseudoarthrosis is identified, revision fusion may be performed concurrently.

While technically less demanding than the index procedure, hardware removal still requires precision to avoid complications such as nerve root injury or dural tears.

Postoperative Care and Recovery

Postoperative management is often less intensive than after the initial fusion surgery. Most patients can mobilize within 24 hours and are discharged within 1–2 days if no complications arise.

- Pain control: Opioids, NSAIDs, and muscle relaxants as appropriate
- Activity restriction: Limited bending, lifting, or twisting for several weeks
- Physical therapy: Introduced based on patient needs and fusion status
- Follow-up imaging: Performed to ensure continued spinal stability

Recovery time is generally shorter than after initial fusion, with most patients returning to light activities within 2–4 weeks (Burneikiene et al., 2015).

Outcomes of Hardware Removal

Outcomes following hardware removal are mixed and depend heavily on patient selection. In patients with hardware-related pain and confirmed solid fusion, removal may lead to significant symptom relief. However, in other cases, pain may persist or worsen due to other underlying conditions such as adjacent segment disease or incomplete fusion.

A study by Campbell et al. (2013) reported that approximately 60–70% of patients experienced improvement in pain after removal, particularly those with prominent hardware or confirmed solid fusion. However, the same study noted a 20% complication rate, highlighting the importance of appropriate indication and surgical planning.

Complications and Risks

Like all surgical procedures, hardware removal carries risks. Common complications include:

- Neurologic injury
- Dural tear and cerebrospinal fluid (CSF) leak
- Infection
- Bleeding
- Recurrent instability if the fusion is incomplete
- No improvement in symptoms

Reoperation in the presence of dense fibrosis or inadequate bony fusion increases the likelihood of complications (Glassman et al., 2006).

Contraindications to Hardware Removal

Hardware removal is generally contraindicated in the following scenarios:

- Incomplete fusion (pseudoarthrosis) without concurrent revision fusion
- Severe osteoporosis, which may be exacerbated by implant removal
- Absence of clear hardware-related symptoms

In these situations, removal may lead to spinal instability, deformity progression, or persistent symptoms.

Conclusion

Hardware removal following lumbar spinal fusion is a selective procedure best reserved for patients with specific, well-defined indications. Although many patients may experience symptomatic relief, particularly in cases of confirmed solid fusion and hardware irritation, outcomes are not universally positive. Careful preoperative evaluation and patient counseling are essential. Surgeons should be vigilant for complications and prepared to revise or extend fusion if necessary.

Chapter 25
Support Groups for Back Pain: The Psychological, Mental and Emotional side

Introduction

Chronic back pain is a widespread health condition that affects millions of individuals worldwide and often extends beyond physical discomfort. While medical treatments focus on reducing pain and improving mobility, the psychological, mental, and emotional effects of long-term back pain are frequently overlooked. Individuals with chronic back pain commonly experience depression, anxiety, stress, and social isolation. Support groups have become an important complementary resource that addresses these non-physical aspects of pain by providing emotional validation, coping strategies, and a sense of community.

Psychological Impact of Chronic Back Pain

Living with persistent back pain can significantly affect an individual's psychological well-being. Research shows that chronic pain is strongly associated with increased rates of depression and anxiety due to ongoing discomfort, reduced independence, and limitations in daily activities (Gatchel et al., 2007). Feelings of helplessness and frustration may develop when pain persists despite treatment, leading to negative thought patterns and decreased self-efficacy. Support groups help counter these psychological effects by allowing individuals to share experiences with others who understand their struggles, which can reduce feelings of hopelessness and promote a more positive mindset.

Mental Health Benefits of Support Groups

Support groups provide a structured environment where individuals with back pain can openly discuss their challenges without fear of judgment. This shared experience can normalize emotional reactions to chronic pain and reduce mental distress. Studies suggest that participation in pain-related support groups can improve coping skills, increase emotional resilience, and enhance perceived control over pain (Turk & Okifuji, 2002). Group discussions often introduce cognitive and behavioral strategies, such as relaxation techniques and positive reframing, which can help individuals better manage pain-related stress.

Emotional Support and Social Connection

Emotionally, chronic back pain can be isolating, as sufferers may feel misunderstood by friends, family, or coworkers who do not experience daily pain. Support groups address this emotional burden by fostering empathy, trust, and mutual encouragement. Emotional validation from peers can reduce loneliness and increase feelings of belonging, which are essential for emotional health. Research indicates that social support plays a critical role in reducing emotional distress and improving overall quality of life among individuals with chronic pain (McCracken & Vowles, 2014).

Role of Support Groups in Pain Coping

Support groups also encourage adaptive coping mechanisms that improve emotional regulation. By learning from others' experiences, individuals may develop healthier ways to respond to pain flare-ups and emotional setbacks. The emotional empowerment gained from group participation can lead to increased motivation, improved mood, and greater acceptance of pain as a manageable condition rather than a defining limitation. This emotional shift can positively influence pain perception and mental health outcomes.

Conclusion

Support groups play a vital role in addressing the psychological, mental, and emotional challenges associated with chronic back pain. Beyond physical symptoms, back pain affects emotional well-being, mental health, and social functioning. Support groups provide a safe space for emotional expression, shared understanding, and the development of effective coping strategies. When combined with medical treatment, participation in support groups can significantly improve emotional resilience, mental health, and overall quality of life for individuals living with chronic back pain.

Chapter 26
The Journey Continues...

Introduction

Low back pain is often described as a physical condition, but for those who live with it daily, it becomes a journey that affects every aspect of life. My experience with low back pain has been ongoing, unpredictable, and at times overwhelming. What began as a physical issue gradually evolved into a challenge that tested my mental strength, emotional resilience, and sense of identity. This essay reflects on my personal journey with low back pain and explores how adaptation, self-awareness, and emotional growth have become essential parts of continuing forward.

Living With Daily Pain

Living with low back pain means constantly adjusting to limitations that others may not see or understand. Simple activities such as sitting for long periods, standing, or even sleeping can become painful obstacles. There are days when the pain is manageable and days when it feels consuming. This unpredictability has required me to become more aware of my body and its signals. Over time, I have learned that pacing myself and listening to my physical limits is not a weakness, but a necessity.

Emotional and Mental Challenges

Beyond the physical discomfort, low back pain has had a significant emotional and mental impact. Frustration often arises when pain interferes with responsibilities, goals, or social activities. At times, I have experienced feelings of sadness, anxiety, and isolation, particularly when others struggle to understand the invisible nature of chronic pain. Research shows that chronic pain is closely linked to emotional distress and mental health challenges, including depression and anxiety (Gatchel et al., 2007). Recognizing this connection helped me understand that my emotional reactions were valid responses to a difficult situation, not personal failures.

Growth Through Adaptation

As my journey with low back pain continues, adaptation has become a central theme. I have learned to redefine productivity and success based on what my body allows rather than what I expect from myself. This shift in mindset has been empowering. Developing coping strategies such as gentle movement, rest, and stress management has helped me regain a sense of control. Emotionally, learning to practice patience and self-compassion has been just as important as managing the physical pain.

Support and Self-Acceptance

Support from others has played a meaningful role in my journey. Whether through healthcare providers, support groups, or understanding individuals, having validation and encouragement has reduced feelings of isolation. Accepting that low back pain is part of my life — rather than something that defines me — has been a turning point. Acceptance does not mean giving up; instead, it means acknowledging reality while continuing to move forward with resilience and hope.

Conclusion

The journey with low back pain is ongoing and ever-changing. While the pain itself may not disappear, my response to it has evolved. Through self-awareness, emotional growth, and adaptation, I have learned that healing is not only physical but also mental and emotional. My journey continues, not despite low back pain, but alongside it, shaped by strength, perseverance, and the determination to live a meaningful life.

My question now is whether removing all the hardware in my back is the right next step. As of February 6, 2026, while the pain has lessened, I continue to experience constant and significant discomfort. Seven days a week, I rely on ice during the day and heat at night—measures that only mask the symptoms rather than address the underlying problem.

Removing the hardware offers no guarantee that the discomfort will improve and carries the risk that pain could return. I wrestle with this decision daily: do I accept living this way indefinitely, or do I take the risk in hopes of finding relief? I fear the worst but continue to hope for the best.

I don't believe patients should be left to navigate decisions like this without clearer guidance, greater certainty, and deeper trust in the medical process. I hope that emerging technologies, artificial intelligence, and future innovations will offer better answers and renewed hope.

For now, the future feels uncertain—and that is where this chapter rests. Only time will reveal how my journey unfolds, but I sincerely hope that yours leads to healing, progress, and success. Back pain is truly crippling and should never take away our ability to live fully, love deeply, and enjoy life.

Update

Since 2020, I have been on a difficult journey of my own with chronic low back pain. From injections and medications to four unsuccessful surgeries and countless other treatments, the list continues on.

As of June 2026, I am preparing for a second attempt at a spinal cord stimulator, hopeful that it may provide some much-needed relief.

Living with constant pain has affected so many aspects of my life. There are days when it is difficult to enjoy time with family, loss of work in my field of law enforcement, focus on advocacy, or simply do the things I love. Yet, like so many others facing their own battles, I continue to move forward one day at a time.

I am hopeful for better days ahead and grateful for every bit of support, encouragement, and understanding along the way. Thank you for always taking the time to listen and for standing beside me during this journey.

We will see what the future holds, but I remain determined to keep fighting.

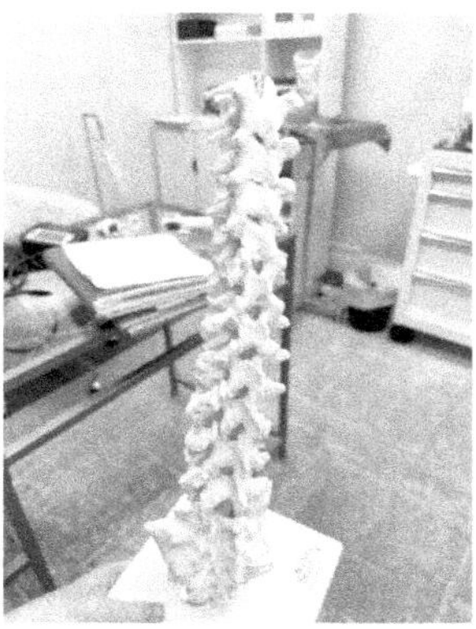

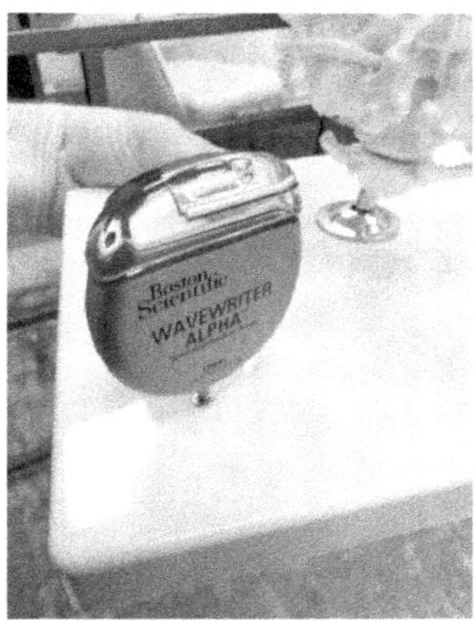

Legal Disclaimer

This book is not intended to provide medical advice in any way and is not meant to replace seeking a certified medical professional. It is only a guide on my individual encounters with my own medical journey and battling my low back pain. ***This book is for educational and informational purposes only.***

Please seek a state certified/licensed medical doctor/professional in your state for any and all medical advice.

About the Author

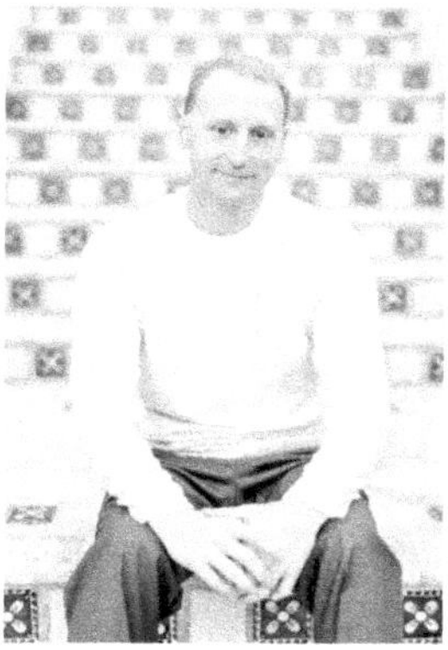

More about Dr. George Ackerman

Dr. George M. Ackerman is a college professor in criminal justice, business, and law. He received his Ph.D. from the School of Public Service Leadership, Capella University; J.D. from the Shepard Broad Law Center, Nova Southeastern University; and police certification from Miami-Dade College School of Justice. His current energy is focused on advocating for a cure for Parkinson's disease through a wide range of avenues and outreach activities.

Dr. Ackerman has participated in numerous charity events; has addressed community, governmental, and international groups; has interviewed people living with Parkinson's, researchers, and advocates; has given interviews; has written about his experiences; and has participated in and conducted seminars, with plans for continued and additional activities. He also leads support groups on caregiving and loss.

Dr. Ackerman founded https://www.togetherforsharon.com/ in memory of his mother, Sharon Riff Ackerman, to increase Parkinson's awareness and research toward a cure. His dedicated interest in and passion for this work to ensure others never feel alone.

Dr. Ackerman's other interests include running charity 5Ks, basketball, and family time with his wife and three wonderful children.

References

Ablin, J. N., Elkayam, O., Fitzcharles, M. A., & Häuser, W. (2016). The role of cannabinoids in the treatment of rheumatic diseases: A review of the evidence. Seminars in Arthritis and Rheumatism, 45(5), 677–684.

Adams, M. A., Dolan, P., & Hutton, W. C. (2020). Biomechanics of back pain. British Journal of Sports Medicine, 54(2), 69–74.

Abdi, S., Datta, S., Trescot, A. M., Schultz, D. M., Adlaka, R., Atluri, S. L. & Manchikanti, L. (2007). Epidural steroids in the management of chronic spinal pain: a systematic review. Pain Physician, 10(1), 185–212.

Akuthota, V., & Nadler, S. F. (2004). Core strengthening. Archives of Physical Medicine and Rehabilitation, 85(3), S86–S92.

Andrade, N. S., Flynn, J. P., Bartanusz, V., Whitmore, R. G., & Witham, T. F. (2015). Hospital volume and complications after elective lumbar spinal fusion: A study of 237,363 patients. Spine, 40(13), 1110–1117.

Bair, M. J., Robinson, R. L., Katon, W., & Kroenke, K. (2003). Depression and pain comorbidity: A literature review. Archives of Internal Medicine, 163(20), 2433–2445.

Balagué, F., Mannion, A. F., Pellisé, F., & Cedraschi, C. (2012). Non-specific low back pain. The Lancet, 379(9814), 482–491.

Benzon, H. T., Huntoon, M. A., & Rathmell, J. P. (2015). Improving the safety of epidural steroid injections. Journal of the American Medical Association, 313(17), 1713–1714.

Benyamin, R. M., Manchikanti, L., Parr, A. T., Diwan, S., Singh, V., Falco, F. J. E., ... & Hirsch, J. A. (2012). The effectiveness of lumbar interlaminar epidural injections in managing chronic low back and lower extremity pain. Pain Physician, 15(4), E363–E404.

Bishop, P. A., Jones, E., & Woods, A. K. (2017). Recovery from training: A brief review. Journal of Strength and Conditioning Research, 22(3), 1015–1024.

Block, A. R., Gatchel, R. J., Deardorff, W. W., & Guyer, R. D. (2001). The psychology of spine surgery. American Psychological Association.

Brinjikji, W., Luetmer, P. H., Comstock, B., Bresnahan, B. W., Chen, L. E., Deyo, R. A., & Jarvik, J. G. (2015). Systematic literature review of imaging features of spinal degeneration in asymptomatic populations. AJNR. American Journal of Neuroradiology, 36(4), 811–816.

Brox, J. I., Reikeras, O., Nygaard, O., Sorensen, R., Indahl, A., Holm, I. & Keller, A. (2003). Lumbar instrumented fusion compared with cognitive intervention and exercises in patients with chronic low back pain after previous surgery for disc herniation: A prospective randomized controlled study. Pain, 105(1-2), 77–85.

Buchbinder, R., Osborne, R. H., Ebeling, P. R., Wark, J. D., & Mitchell, P. (2009). A randomized trial of vertebroplasty for painful osteoporotic vertebral fractures. New England Journal of Medicine, 361(6), 557–568.

Burneikiene, S., Nelson, E. L., Mason, A., & Villavicencio, A. T. (2015). Complications in elective spine surgery patients 65 years of age and older: An analysis of spine surgery complications and perioperative events. Surgical Neurology International, 6(Suppl 5), S140–S149.

Campbell, P. G., Yadla, S., Nasser, R., Malone, J., Maltenfort, M. G., Harrop, J. S., & Ratliff, J. K. (2013). Early complications related to approach in thoracic and lumbar spine surgery: A single center prospective study. World Neurosurgery, 79(1), 107–113.

Chan, C. W., & Peng, P. (2011). Failed back surgery syndrome. Pain Medicine, 12(4), 577–606.

Cherkin, D. C., Sherman, K. J., Balderson, B. H., Cook, A. J., Anderson, M. L., Hawkes, R. J., Hansen, K. E., & Turner, J. A. (2016). Effect of mindfulness-based stress reduction vs cognitive behavioral therapy or usual care on back pain and functional limitations in adults with chronic low back pain. JAMA, 315(12), 1240–1249.

Chou, R., Baisden, J., Carragee, E. J., Resnick, D. K., Shaffer, W. O., & Loeser, J. D. (2009). Surgery for low back pain: A review of the evidence for an American Pain Society Clinical Practice Guideline. Spine, 34(10), 1094–1109.

Chou, R., Deyo, R., Friedly, J., Skelly, A., Hashimoto, R., Weimer, M. & Fu, R. (2015). Systemic pharmacologic therapies for low back pain: A systematic review for an American College of Physicians clinical practice guideline. Annals of Internal Medicine, 166(7), 480–492.

Chou, R., Hashimoto, R., Friedly, J., Fu, R., Dana, T., Sullivan, S. D., & Brodt, E. D. (2015). Pain management injection therapies for low back pain. Agency for Healthcare Research and Quality (US).

Chou, R., Hashimoto, R., Friedly, J., Fu, R., Dana, T., Sullivan, S. D. & Deyo, R. A. (2017). Noninvasive treatments for low back pain. Agency for Healthcare Research and Quality.

Chou, R., Qaseem, A., Snow, V., Casey, D., Cross, J. T., Shekelle, P., & Owens, D. K. (2011). Diagnosis and treatment of low back pain: A joint clinical practice guideline from the American College of Physicians and the American Pain Society. Annals of Internal Medicine, 147(7), 478–491.

Clark, W., Bird, P., Gonski, P., Diamond, T., Smerdely, P., McNeil, H., & Chung, J. (2016). Safety and efficacy of vertebroplasty for acute painful osteoporotic fractures (VAPOUR): a multicentre, randomised, double-blind, placebo-controlled trial. The Lancet, 388(10052), 1408–1416.

Cohen, S. P., Hurley, R. W., Buckenmaier, C. C., Kurihara, C., Morlion, B., & Wu, C. L. (2008). Pain management best practices. Pain Medicine, 9(2), 214–228.

Cohen, S. P., Kennedy, D. J., Dragovich, A., Kapural, L., MacVicar, J., Schultz, D. M., & Vorobeychik, Y. (2020). Evidence-based interventions for low back pain. Best Practice & Research Clinical Anaesthesiology, 34(3), 277–292.

Compston, J., McClung, M., & Leslie, W. (2019). Osteoporosis. The Lancet, 393(10169), 364–376.

Cosman, F., de Beur, S. J., LeBoff, M. S., Lewiecki, E. M., Tanner, B., Randall, S., & Lindsay, R. (2014). Clinician's guide to prevention and treatment of osteoporosis. Osteoporosis International, 25(10), 2359–2381.

Cruz-Díaz, D., Lomas-Vega, R., Osuna-Pérez, M. C., Hita-Contreras, F., & Martínez-Amat, A. (2015). Effects of core stability training on dynamic balance and trunk endurance in professional soccer players. Physical Therapy in Sport, 16(4), 349–354.

Deer, T. R., Mekhail, N., Provenzano, D., Pope, J. E., Krames, E. S., Leong, M. & North, R. B. (2014). The appropriate use of neurostimulation of the spinal cord and peripheral nervous system for the treatment of chronic pain and ischemic diseases: the Neuromodulation Appropriateness Consensus Committee. Neuromodulation: Technology at the Neural Interface, 17(6), 515-550.

Delitto, A., George, S. Z., Van Dillen, L. R., Whitman, J. M., Sowa, G., Shekelle, P. & Godges, J. J. (2012). Low back pain. Journal of Orthopaedic & Sports Physical Therapy, 42(4), A1–A57.

Deyo, R. A. (2002). Diagnostic evaluation of LBP: reaching a specific diagnosis is often impossible. Archives of Internal Medicine, 162(13), 1444–1447.

Deyo, R. A., Mirza, S. K., & Martin, B. I. (2010). Back pain prevalence and visit rates: Estimates from U.S. national surveys, 2002. Spine, 31(23), 2724–2727.

Deyo, R. A., Mirza, S. K., Martin, B. I., Kreuter, W., Goodman, D. C., & Jarvik, J. G. (2010). Trends, major medical complications, and charges associated with surgery for lumbar spinal stenosis in older adults. JAMA, 303(13), 1259–1265.

Deyo, R. A., Mirza, S. K., Turner, J. A., & Martin, B. I. (2010). Overtreating chronic back pain: time to back off? Journal of the American Board of Family Medicine, 22(1), 62–68.

Deyo, R. A., Von Korff, M., & Duhrkoop, D. (2015). Opioids for low back pain. BMJ, 350, g6380.

Deyo, R. A., & Weinstein, J. N. (2001). Low back pain. New England Journal of Medicine, 344(5), 363–370.

Dowell, D., Haegerich, T. M., & Chou, R. (2016). CDC guideline for prescribing opioids for chronic pain—United States, 2016. JAMA, 315(15), 1624–1645.

Ehde, D. M., Dillworth, T. M., & Turner, J. A. (2014). Cognitive-behavioral therapy for individuals with chronic pain: Efficacy, innovations, and directions for research. American Psychologist, 69(2), 153–166.

Enke, O., New, H. A., New, C. H., Mathieson, S., McLachlan, A. J., Latimer, J., ... & Maher, C. G. (2018). Anticonvulsants in the treatment of low back pain and lumbar radicular pain: A systematic review and meta-analysis. CMAJ, 190(26), E786–E793.

Fairbank, J., Frost, H., Wilson-MacDonald, J., Yu, L. M., Barker, K., & Collins, R. (2005). Randomized controlled trial to compare surgical stabilization of the lumbar spine with an intensive rehabilitation program for patients with chronic low back pain: The MRC Spine Stabilization Trial. BMJ, 330(7502), 1233.

Farrokhi, F. R., Lebrun, C. T., Tighe, P. J., & Kiester, P. D. (2017). High surgical volume and outcomes for spinal fusion. Spine, 42(17), 1307–1315.

Fink, H. A., Milavetz, D. L., Palermo, L., Nevitt, M. C., Cauley, J. A., & Ensrud, K. E. (2003). What proportion of incident radiographic vertebral deformities is clinically diagnosed and vice versa? Journal of Bone and Mineral Research, 20(7), 1216–1222.

Foster, N. E., Anema, J. R., Cherkin, D., Chou, R., Cohen, S. P., Gross, D. P. & Maher, C. G. (2018). Prevention and treatment of low back pain: Evidence, challenges, and promising directions. The Lancet, 391(10137), 2368–2383.

Fritzell, P., Hägg, O., Wessberg, P., & Nordwall, A. (2001). 2001 Volvo Award Winner in Clinical Studies: Lumbar fusion versus nonsurgical treatment for chronic low back pain. Spine, 26(23), 2521–2532.

Furlan, A. D., van Tulder, M. W., Cherkin, D. C., Tsukayama, H., Lao, L., Koes, B. W., & Berman, B. M. (2003). Acupuncture and dry-needling for low back pain: An updated systematic review within the framework of the Cochrane Collaboration. Spine, 28(15), 1527–1537.

Gajraj, N. M. (2005). Transforaminal epidural steroid injections. Current Pain and Headache Reports, 9(1), 37–43.

Gatchel, R. J., McGeary, D. D., McGeary, C. A., & Lippe, B. (2014). Interdisciplinary chronic pain management: Past, present, and future. American Psychologist, 69(2), 119–130.

Gatchel, R. J., Peng, Y. B., Peters, M. L., Fuchs, P. N., & Turk, D. C. (2007). The biopsychosocial approach to chronic pain: Scientific advances and future directions. *Psychological Bulletin, 133*(4), 581–624.

Gatti, A., Sabato, A. F., Occhioni, R., & Reale, C. (2016). Analgesic effect of a lidocaine patch in patients with chronic low back pain. Current Medical Research and Opinion, 28(6), 1005–1012.

GBD 2017 Disease and Injury Incidence and Prevalence Collaborators. (2018). Global, regional, and national incidence, prevalence, and years lived with disability for 354 diseases and injuries for 195 countries and territories, 1990–2017. The Lancet, 392(10159), 1789–1858.

Geneen, L. J., Moore, R. A., Clarke, C., Martin, D., Colvin, L. A., & Smith, B. H. (2017). Physical activity and exercise for chronic pain in adults: An overview of Cochrane Reviews. Cochrane Database of Systematic Reviews, 2017(4), CD011279.

Glassman, S. D., Alegre, G., Carreon, L., Dimar, J. R., & Johnson, J. R. (2006). Perioperative complications of lumbar instrumentation and fusion in older adults. Spine, 31(14), 1575–1580.

Gold, D. T., & Silverman, S. L. (2016). The pain and impact of vertebral fractures from osteoporosis. American Journal of Medicine, 129(2), 95–103.

Gronlund, C., Öhlin, A., & Magnusson, M. (2021). Second opinion in spine surgery: A prospective observational study in a university hospital. BMC Health Services Research, 21(1), 1125.

Guyer, R. D., McAfee, P. C., Banco, R. J., Bitan, F. D., Cappuccino, A., Geisler, F. H. Blumenthal, S. L. (2009). Prospective, randomized, multicenter Food and Drug Administration investigational device exemptions study of lumbar total disc replacement with the CHARITÉ artificial disc versus lumbar fusion: Five-year follow-up. Spine Journal, 9(5), 374–386.

Hall, A. M., Kamper, S. J., & Maher, C. G. (2016). Does pain-catastrophising mediate the effect of Tai Chi on treatment outcomes for people with low back pain? Complementary Therapies in Medicine, 25, 61–66.

Hartvigsen, J., Hancock, M. J., Kongsted, A., Louw, Q., Ferreira, M. L., Genevay, S. (2018). What low back pain is and why we need to pay attention. The Lancet, 391(10137), 2356–2367.

Hayden, J. A., Ellis, J., Ogilvie, R., Stewart, S. A., Bagg, M. K., Stanojevic, S., & Yamato, T. P. (2021). Exercise therapy for chronic low back pain: A systematic review of treatment effectiveness. BMJ Open, 11(9), e053497.

Henschke, N., Ostelo, R. W., van Tulder, M. W., Vlaeyen, J. W., Morley, S., Assendelft, W. J., & Main, C. J. (2010). Behavioral treatment for chronic low-back pain. Cochrane Database of Systematic Reviews, 2010(7), CD002014.

Hodges, P. W. (2003). Core stability exercise in chronic low back pain. Orthopedic Clinics of North America, 34(2), 245–254.

Hodges, P. W., & Richardson, C. A. (1996). Inefficient muscular stabilization of the lumbar spine associated with low back pain: A motor control evaluation of transversus abdominis. Spine, 21(22), 2640–2650.

Hoffman, B. M., Papas, R. K., Chatkoff, D. K., & Kerns, R. D. (2007). Meta-analysis of psychological interventions for chronic low back pain. Health Psychology, 26(1), 1–9.

Hoy, D., March, L., Brooks, P., Blyth, F., Woolf, A., Bain, C. & Buchbinder, R. (2014). The global burden of low back pain: Estimates from the Global Burden of Disease 2010 study. Annals of the Rheumatic Diseases, 73(6), 968–974.

Hoy, D., Bain, C., Williams, G., March, L., Brooks, P., Blyth, F. & Buchbinder, R. (2012). A systematic review of the global prevalence of low back pain. Arthritis & Rheumatism, 64(6), 2028–2037.

Jarvik, J. G., & Deyo, R. A. (2002). Diagnostic evaluation of low back pain with emphasis on imaging. Annals of Internal Medicine, 137(7), 586–597.

Jensen, M. C., Brant-Zawadzki, M. N., Obuchowski, N., Modic, M. T., Malkasian, D., & Ross, J. S. (1994). Magnetic resonance imaging of the lumbar spine in people without back pain. New England Journal of Medicine, 331(2), 69–73.

Kabat-Zinn, J. (1982). An outpatient program in behavioral medicine for chronic pain patients based on the practice of mindfulness meditation: Theoretical considerations and preliminary results. General Hospital Psychiatry, 4(1), 33–47.

Kamper, S. J., Apeldoorn, A. T., Chiarotto, A., Smeets, R. J., Ostelo, R. W., Guzman, J. & van Tulder, M. W. (2015). Multidisciplinary biopsychosocial rehabilitation for chronic low back pain. Cochrane Database of Systematic Reviews, 2015(9), CD000963.

Kanis, J. A., Cooper, C., Rizzoli, R., Reginster, J. Y., & Scientific Advisory Board of the European Society for Clinical and Economic Aspects of Osteoporosis and Osteoarthritis (ESCEO) and the Committees of Scientific Advisors and National Societies of the International Osteoporosis Foundation (IOF). (2019). European guidance for the diagnosis and management of osteoporosis in postmenopausal women. Osteoporosis International, 30(1), 3–44.

Katz, J. N. (2006). Lumbar disc disorders and low-back pain: Socioeconomic factors and consequences. The Journal of Bone and Joint Surgery. American Volume, 88(suppl_2), 21–24.

Kim, D. Y., Lee, S. H., Chung, S. K., & Lee, H. Y. (2012). Removal of instrumentation after successful posterior lumbar interbody fusion using cages and pedicle screws. Spine, 27(8), 871–876.

Krebs, E. E., Gravely, A., Nugent, S., Jensen, A. C., DeRonne, B., Goldsmith, E. S. & Noorbaloochi, S. (2018). Effect of opioid vs nonopioid medications on pain-related function in patients with chronic back pain or hip or knee osteoarthritis pain: The SPACE randomized clinical trial. JAMA, 319(9), 872–882.

Kumar, K., Taylor, R. S., Jacques, L., Eldabe, S., Meglio, M., Molet, J. & North, R. B. (2007). Spinal cord stimulation versus conventional medical management for neuropathic pain: a multicentre randomised controlled trial in patients with failed back surgery syndrome. Pain, 132(1-2), 179-188.

Lentz, T. A., Beneciuk, J. M., & George, S. Z. (2022). Reducing unnecessary spine surgery: The role of second opinions in musculoskeletal care. Health Affairs, 41(3), 415–421.

Louw, A., Diener, I., Butler, D. S., & Puentedura, E. J. (2011). The effect of neuroscience education on pain, disability, anxiety, and stress in chronic musculoskeletal pain. Archives of Physical Medicine and Rehabilitation, 92(12), 2041–2056.

MacDonald, D. A., Fernández-de-las-Peñas, C., & Flynn, T. (2019). Low back pain and fear avoidance. Manual Therapy, 24(2), 177–184.

Maher, C., Underwood, M., & Buchbinder, R. (2017). Non-specific low back pain. The Lancet, 389(10070), 736–747.

Main, C. J., Foster, N., & Buchbinder, R. (2010). How important are back pain beliefs and expectations for satisfactory recovery from back pain? Best Practice & Research Clinical Rheumatology, 24(2), 205–217.

Manchikanti, L., Boswell, M. V., Datta, S., Fellows, B., & Abdi, S. (2013). Comprehensive review of therapeutic interventions in managing chronic spinal pain. Pain Physician, 12(4), E123–E198.

Manchikanti, L., Boswell, M. V., Singh, V., Pampati, V., Damron, K. S., & Beyer, C. (2003). Prevalence of facet joint pain in chronic spinal pain of cervical, thoracic, and lumbar regions. BMC Musculoskeletal Disorders, 5, 15.

Manchikanti, L., Falco, F. J., Benyamin, R. M., & Hirsch, J. A. (2012). Efficacy of transforaminal epidural injections in managing lumbar disc herniation and radiculopathy. Pain Physician, 15(3), E199–E245.

Manchikanti, L., Singh, V., Kloth, D. S., Slipman, C. W., Jasper, J. F., & Trescot, A. M. (2009). Comprehensive review of epidemiology, scope, and impact of spinal pain. Pain Physician, 12(4), E35–E70.

Martin, B. I., Mirza, S. K., Comstock, B. A., Gray, D. T., Kreuter, W., & Deyo, R. A. (2007). Reoperation rates following lumbar spine surgery and the influence of spinal fusion procedures. Spine, 32(3), 382–387.

Martinez-Calderon, J., Flores-Cortes, M., Morales-Asencio, J. M., Luque-Suarez, A. (2018). Which biopsychosocial factors are associated with pain in individuals with chronic non-specific low back pain? A cross-sectional study. Pain Medicine, 19(11), 2336–2346.

McCracken, L. M., & Vowles, K. E. (2014). Acceptance and commitment therapy and mindfulness for chronic pain: Model, process, and progress. *American Psychologist, 69*(2), 178–187.McGill, S. M. (2016). Back mechanic: The secrets to a healthy spine your doctor isn't telling you. Backfitpro Inc.

Melzack, R., & Wall, P. D. (1965). Pain mechanisms: a new theory. Science, 150(3699), 971-979.

Morley, S., Eccleston, C., & Williams, A. (1999). Systematic review and meta-analysis of randomized controlled trials of cognitive behavior therapy and behavior therapy for chronic pain in adults, excluding headache. Pain, 80(1–2), 1–13.

National Osteoporosis Foundation. (2023). Osteoporosis fast facts. https://www.nof.org

Nicholas, M. K., Asghari, A., & Blyth, F. M. (2011). What do the numbers mean? Normative data in chronic pain measures. Pain, 152(6), 1045–1049.

Nicholas, M. K., Linton, S. J., Watson, P. J., & Main, C. J. (2011). Early identification and management of psychological risk factors ("yellow flags") in patients with low back pain: a reappraisal. Physical Therapy, 91(5), 737–753.

North, R. B., Kidd, D. H., Farrokhi, F., & Piantadosi, S. A. (2011). Spinal cord stimulation versus repeated lumbosacral spine surgery for chronic pain: a randomized, controlled trial. Neurosurgery, 56(1), 98-106.

Orenstein, E. W., Pritchard, J., & Duda, N. (2020). The impact of second opinions in spine surgery: A systematic review. Spine, 45(23), E1603–E1611.

O'Sullivan, P. B., Caneiro, J. P., O'Keeffe, M., & O'Sullivan, K. (2015). Cognitive functional therapy: An integrated behavioral approach for the targeted management of disabling low back pain. Physical Therapy, 95(5), 730–738.

Page, P., Frank, C. C., & Lardner, R. (2012). Assessment and treatment of muscle imbalance: The Janda approach. Human Kinetics.

Paige, N. M., Miake-Lye, I. M., Booth, M. S., Beroes, J. M., Mardian, A. S., Dougherty, P. & Shekelle, P. G. (2017). Association of spinal manipulative therapy with clinical benefit and harm for acute low back pain: Systematic review and meta-analysis. JAMA, 317(14), 1451–1460.

Panjabi, M. M. (1992). The stabilizing system of the spine. Part I. Function, dysfunction, adaptation, and enhancement. Journal of Spinal Disorders, 5(4), 383–389.

Pincus, T., Burton, A. K., Vogel, S., & Field, A. P. (2002). A systematic review of psychological factors as predictors of chronicity/disability in prospective cohorts of low back pain. Spine, 27(5), E109–E120.

Pinheiro, M. B., Ferreira, M. L., Refshauge, K., Ordoñana, J. R., Machado, G. C., Prado, L. R., & Ferreira, P. H. (2016). Symptoms of depression and risk of new episodes of low back pain: A systematic review and meta-analysis. Arthritis Care & Research, 68(9), 1313–1321.

Qaseem, A., Wilt, T. J., McLean, R. M., & Forciea, M. A. (2017). Noninvasive treatments for acute, subacute, and chronic low back pain: A clinical practice guideline. Annals of Internal Medicine, 166(7), 514–530.

Ropper, A. H., & Zafonte, R. D. (2015). Diagnosis and management of back pain. The New England Journal of Medicine, 372(6), 553–560.

Searle, A., Spink, M., Ho, A., & Chuter, V. (2015). Exercise interventions for the treatment of chronic low back pain: A systematic review and meta-analysis of randomized controlled trials. Clinical Rehabilitation, 29(12), 1155–1167.

Shamsi, M. B., Sarrafzadeh, J., Jamshidi, A. A., & Karimi, A. (2015). Comparison of lumbopelvic stability and muscle activation patterns in people with and without chronic low back pain: A cross-sectional study. Journal of Physical Therapy Science, 27(4), 1091–1096.

Sherman, K. J., Cherkin, D. C., Wellman, R. D., Cook, A. J., Hawkes, R. J., Delaney, K., & Deyo, R. A. (2011). A randomized trial comparing yoga, stretching, and a self-care book for chronic low back pain. Archives of Internal Medicine, 171(22), 2019–2026.

Shiri, R., Falah-Hassani, K., & Viikari-Juntura, E. (2018). The effect of physical activity on the incidence of low back pain: A systematic review and meta-analysis. American Journal of Epidemiology, 187(5), 1093–1101.

Shiri, R., Karppinen, J., Leino-Arjas, P., Solovieva, S., & Viikari-Juntura, E. (2010). The association between smoking and low back pain: A meta-analysis. American Journal of Medicine, 123(1), 87.e7 –87.e35.

Sinaki, M. (2017). Musculoskeletal issues in osteoporosis. Current Osteoporosis Reports, 15(5), 333–339.

Standaert, C. J., & Herring, S. A. (2007). Expert opinion and controversies in musculoskeletal and sports medicine: The lumbar spine. Archives of Physical Medicine and Rehabilitation, 88(3), 407–411.

Steffens, D., Maher, C. G., Pereira, L. S., Stevens, M. L., Oliveira, V. C., Chapple, M., & Hancock, M. J. (2016). Prevention of low back pain: A systematic review and meta-analysis. JAMA Internal Medicine, 176(2), 199–208.

Synnott, A., O'Keeffe, M., Bunzli, S., Dankaerts, W., O'Sullivan, P., & O'Sullivan, K. (2015). Physiotherapists may stigmatise or feel unprepared to treat people with low back pain and psychosocial factors that influence recovery: a systematic review. Journal of Physiotherapy, 61(2), 68–76.

Thompson, S., Ghomrawi, H. M. K., & Kates, S. L. (2021). The burden of failed back surgery syndrome. Orthopedic Clinics, 52(4), 539–547.

Turk, D. C., & Okifuji, A. (2002). Psychological factors in chronic pain: Evolution and revolution. Journal of Consulting and Clinical Psychology, 70(3), 678–690

Turk, D. C., Swanson, K. S., & Tunks, E. R. (2011). Psychological approaches in the treatment of chronic pain patients—when pills, scalpels, and needles are not enough. Canadian Journal of Psychiatry, 53(4), 213–223.

Van Tulder, M. W., Touray, T., Furlan, A. D., Solway, S., & Bouter, L. M. (2006). Muscle relaxants for non-specific low back pain. Cochrane Database of Systematic Reviews, (4).

Van Tulder, M. W., Touray, T., Furlan, A. D., Solway, S., & Bouter, L. M. (2000). Muscle relaxants for nonspecific low back pain: A systematic review within the framework of the Cochrane Collaboration. Spine, 28(17), 1978–1992.

Vickers, A. J., Vertosick, E. A., Lewith, G., MacPherson, H., Foster, N. E., Sherman, K. J. & Linde, K. (2018). Acupuncture for chronic pain: Update of an individual patient data meta-analysis. The Journal of Pain, 19(5), 455–474.

Vlaeyen, J. W., & Linton, S. J. (2000). Fear-avoidance and its consequences in chronic musculoskeletal pain: A state of the art. Pain, 85(3), 317–332.

Vos, T., Flaxman, A. D., Naghavi, M., Lozano, R., Michaud, C., Ezzati, M. & Murray, C. J. L. (2012). Years lived with disability (YLDs) for 1160 sequelae of 289 diseases and injuries, 1990–2010: A systematic analysis. The Lancet, 380(9859), 2163–2196.

Waddell, G., & Burton, A. K. (2001). Occupational health guidelines for the management of low back pain at work: Evidence review. Occupational Medicine, 51(2), 124–135.

Walker, B. F., Muller, R., & Grant, W. D. (2003). Low back pain in Australian adults: prevalence and associated disability. Journal of Manipulative and Physiological Therapeutics, 26(6), 341–345.

Wang, M. Y., Chang, P. Y., & Grossman, J. (2021). Minimally invasive spinal surgery: Clinical evidence and future direction. Neurosurgery, 89(3), 349–364.

Weinstein, J. N., Lurie, J. D., Tosteson, T. D., Hanscom, B., Tosteson, A. N., Blood, E. A. & Herkowitz, H. (2006). Surgical vs. nonoperative treatment for lumbar disk herniation: The Spine Patient Outcomes Research Trial (SPORT): A randomized trial. JAMA, 296(20), 2441–2450.

Weinstein, J. N., Tosteson, T. D., Lurie, J. D., Tosteson, A. N., Blood, E. A., Hanscom, B. & Herkowitz, H. (2008). Surgical versus nonoperative treatment for lumbar spinal stenosis four-year results of the Spine Patient Outcomes Research Trial. Spine, 33(25), 2789–2800.

Williams, C. M., Maher, C. G., McLachlan, A. J., Hancock, M. J., McAuley, J. H., Britt, H., & Blyth, F. M. (2014). Efficacy of paracetamol for acute low-back pain: A double-blind, randomized controlled trial. The Lancet, 384(9954), 1586–1596.

Wong, J. J., Côté, P., Sutton, D. A., Randhawa, K., Yu, H., Varatharajan, S., & Southerst, D. (2019). Clinical practice guidelines for the noninvasive management of low back pain: A systematic review by the Ontario Protocol for Traffic Injury Management (OPTIMa) Collaboration. European Journal of Pain, 21(2), 201–216.

Wu, A., March, L., Zheng, X., Huang, J., Wang, X., Zhao, Y. & Hoy, D. (2020). Global low back pain prevalence and years lived with disability from 1990 to 2017: Estimates from the Global Burden of Disease Study 2017. Annals of Translational Medicine, 8(6), 299.

Yoo, J. S., Kim, K. N., Yoon, D. H., Shin, H. C., & Kim, S. H. (2008). The fate of anterior instrumentation after successful fusion in lumbar spine. Journal of Korean Neurosurgical Society, 44(5), 321–326.

Please support

TogetherForSharon®

https://www.togetherforsharon.com/shop/

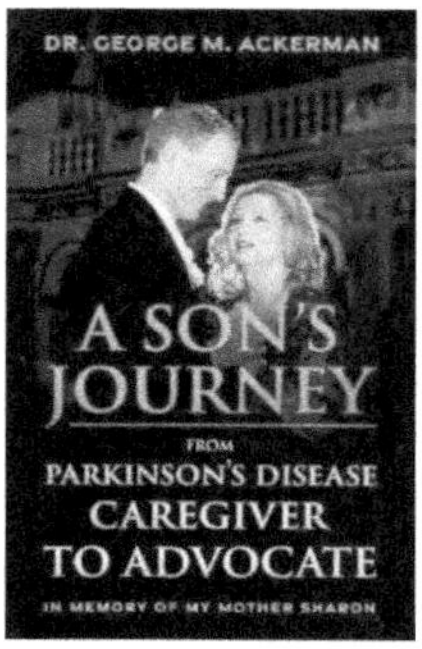

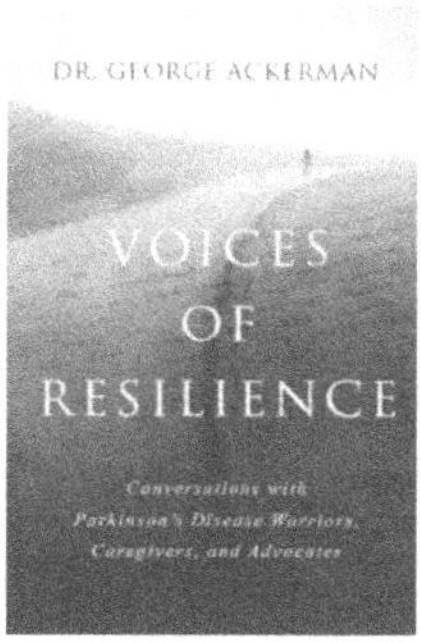

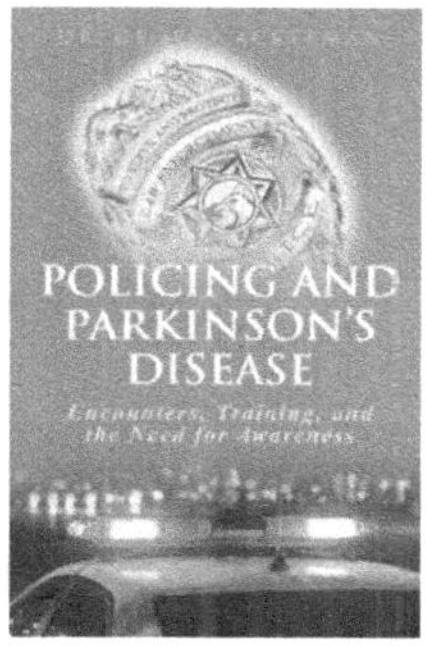

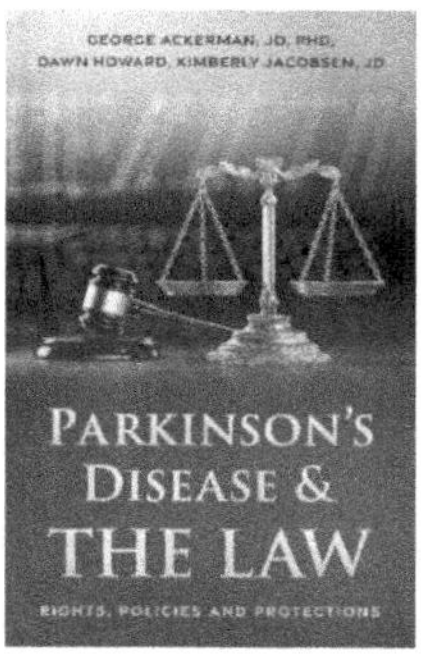

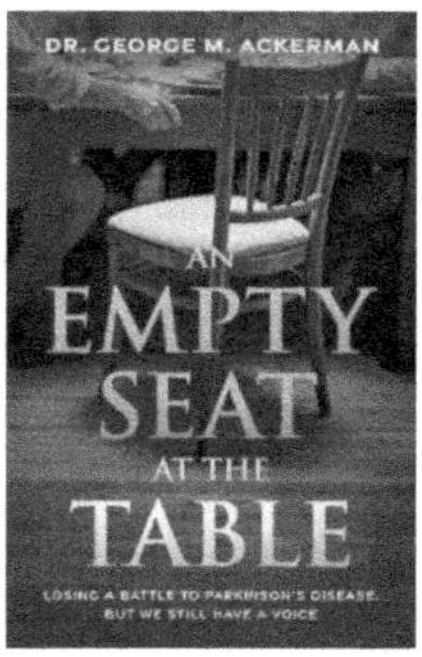

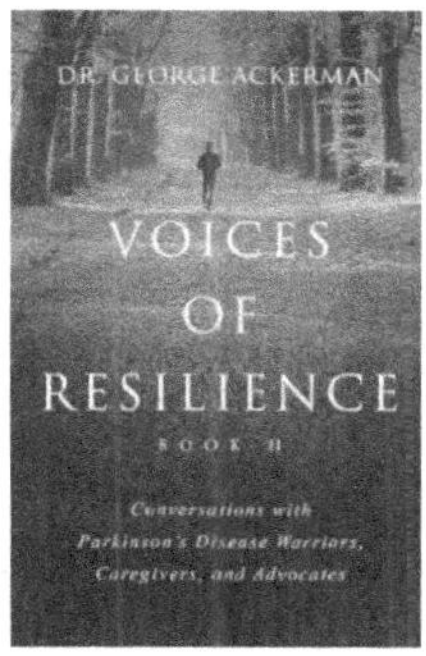

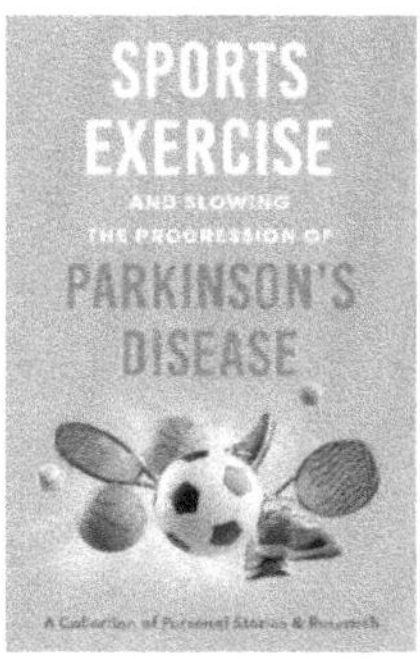

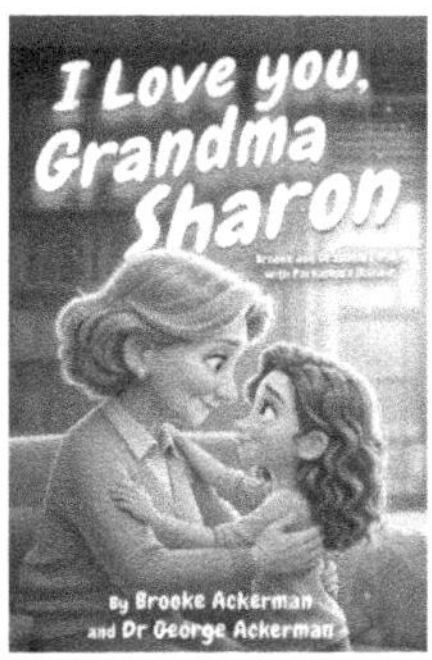

www.ingramcontent.com/pod-product-compliance
Lightning Source LLC
LaVergne TN
LVHW022217200926
848481LV00006B/2004